EVERYDAY

Natural

EVERYDAY
Natural

Jacqueline Ritz

SILOAM

Most CHARISMA HOUSE BOOK GROUP products are available at special quantity discounts for bulk purchase for sales promotions, premiums, fund-raising, and educational needs. For details, write Charisma House Book Group, 600 Rinehart Road, Lake Mary, Florida 32746, or telephone (407) 333-0600.

EVERYDAY NATURAL by Jacqueline Ritz
Published by Siloam
Charisma Media/Charisma House Book Group
600 Rinehart Road
Lake Mary, Florida 32746
www.charismahouse.com

Cover design by Vincent Pirozzi
Design Director: Justin Evans

Visit the author's website at thepaleomama.com; see aslo everydaynaturalbook.com.

Library of Congress Cataloging-in-Publication Data:
Names: Ritz, Jacqueline, author.
Title: Everyday natural / by Jacqueline Ritz.
Description: Lake Mary, Florida : Siloam, [2017] | Includes bibliographical
    references.
Identifiers: LCCN 2017029040| ISBN 9781629991887 (trade paper) | ISBN

9781629991894 (ebook)
Subjects: LCSH: Self-care, Health. | Nutrition. | Weight loss. | Health
  behavior.
Classification: LCC RA776.95 .R583 2017 | DDC 613.2--dc23
LC record available at https://lccn.loc.gov/2017029040

17 18 19 20 21 — 987654321
Printed in the United States of America

In loving memory of my dear sister,
Dinah. Thank you for always believing
in me and bringing so much joy to
my life. You are forever missed.

CONTENTS

RECIPES

PART III

Everyday Home and Garden

PART IV

Everyday Natural Farm

PART V

Everyday Natural Family

ACKNOWLEDGMENTS

I FIND MYSELF HUMBLED by the many people who have provided me with constant support during the last several years.

To my husband, Frank Ritz: thank you for your unwavering care, love, and support as I pursued my dreams. You inspired me to start a blog, and later on you let me bring home chickens! I love you more than anything.

To my mom and best friend, Barbara Dycus: thank you for loving me and raising me to become the woman I am today. Thank you for seeing an opportunity in my work and encouraging me to write a book.

To all my blog readers: you inspire me to keep writing, creating, and sharing this beautiful life with the world.

And lastly, to my Lord and Savior, Jesus Christ: thank You for gathering up the scattered pieces of my life and giving me the courage to create a life that my family and I love.

INTRODUCTION

*I*T SEEMS THAT everyone is talking about natural living today. But why is natural living important? And exactly what is natural living?

There isn't just one simple answer to these questions. What is natural to me or you depends on many things, including the following:

+ Personal circumstances
+ Income
+ Where you live
+ What your dreams are for your family
+ Why you want to live naturally

Big corporations have been jumping on the natural-living bandwagon and labeling their products with terms such as *natural, green,* and *organic.* But not many are actually supporting natural living by spreading the truth about toxic manufacturing practices. The food industry has its own definitions of *natural, green,* and *organic,* and they all fall a bit short of true natural living.

Natural living is all about the choices we make today. Are we choosing to eliminate added chemicals, preservatives, additives, and processing from our lives? Are we choosing "pure" products that are good for us and finding more and more ways to ensure that everything that touches our loved ones is clean? Are we functioning as the security border around our family's life and health?

In this book I want to share how my family and I are choosing to live naturally. Believe me, I'm no expert on the subject, but I have been on the journey to a more natural lifestyle for more than ten years. I have more to learn, but I also have a lot to share about what is and what is not working for us.

I want my book to inspire you to begin your own journey to

natural living. Granted, you may be able to take only a few baby steps right now, but I hope my story and experiences will foster a great big dream in your heart, one that will keep propelling you toward a healthier and more enjoyable lifestyle.

What you read in these pages won't change you unless you catch a vision of how making at least some of the recommended changes will improve the quality of life for you and your family. Most of all, I hope that our story will cause you to dream big about your family's health, and that in this book you will find steps you can use to start living your dream.

> Natural living is all about the choices we make today.

As you will see in the pages that follow, my family and I took very practical steps to adopt a more natural lifestyle. I will tell you more about our journey throughout this book, but just to give you an overview:

1. My husband, Frank, and I spent several years eliminating all the debt we had accumulated so we could live debt-free.

2. We created more family time for ourselves, keeping weekends for family activities and playing games, roughhousing, dancing, singing, and acting foolish together in the evenings.

3. We are limiting the ever-encroaching world of technology to just what we determine is best for us and especially our children. TV time and computer time are limited, and creative playtime is encouraged to spark our children's imaginations.

4. We are constantly doing everything we can to eliminate toxic products from our home and to eat the healthiest, most chemical-free foods we can find and grow ourselves.

5. In 2015 we were able to buy our Gather Heritage Farm, which has more than ten acres for living sustainably and establishing a homestead. This is the fulfillment of our years-long dream, allowing us to grow much of our own food and to raise "heritage" breed animals (traditional breeds farmers raised in the past) for milk and meat, and to breed them for others.

6. Both my husband and I have worked diligently toward the goal of working from home instead of pursuing careers outside the home. We have been fortunate enough to make this dream a reality.

7. We like to call our children "free-range" and are encouraging them to learn from nature and the world all around them.

So, as you begin this book, think about what steps you want to take to realize your own dreams for a better, healthier, more natural lifestyle. Look for ideas in these pages that will help you to take those baby steps forward. And dream big! As you read on, I believe you are going to find some inspiration and information that will get you started on your own journey to a healthy, natural lifestyle.

To make this book as helpful as possible, I have included a list of recommended resources in the appendix. Whenever I mention a natural product or supply that is referenced on that page, it will be marked with an asterisk.

Now that the housekeeping is out of the way, let's begin discovering how to live everyday natural.

Chapter 1

MY JOURNEY BACK
TO NATURAL

I CAN SOMETIMES CLOSE my eyes and smell my childhood. It smells like freshly raked leaves, chlorine on my bathing suit, sweat that lingers on my skin, and freshly popped cheesy popcorn. It tastes like oatmeal cream pies, tacos on a Saturday night, and hose water. I treasure the childhood I had.

I am the middle child. I am the free spirit. My mom said the lyrics of "I Hope You Dance" reminded her of me, and she sang it over me often. I was my daddy's little girl who was willing to hold his hand in mine even when my teenage friends could see.

I would proudly walk beside my big brother, who is huge. Standing over six feet six inches tall, he would stare into the eyes of boys and frighten them away. I'd smile at him because I would rather hang out with him than those stupid boys anyway.

My sister, the youngest of us three, was always my best friend. We loved hard, and we fought even harder. Yet at the end of the day when we lay down in our beds in our shared room, we always said:

"I'm sorry if I've done anything wrong."

"I forgive you. I'm sorry if I've done anything wrong too."

Sometimes we had a line or a blanket dividing our bedroom. Other times we slept in the same bed when outside terrors scared us.

Eventually we grew up.

I started college and then became involved in church ministry. Soon after, I left for Australia, then went to Thailand for a year of missionary work with Youth With a Mission (YWAM). Thailand changed me forever. My passion became showing women how beautiful they are. I talked to prostitutes and taught them English. I helped at a center that gave women a chance to come out of prostitution by choosing to learn a trade. I even paid for women to spend a night having fun and feasting instead of working in bars.

> My physical body could not process all the strange foods, bacteria, and internal parasites, and I became progressively sicker.

But life became hard for me there by myself. I was lonely without the strong support system I'd always had with my family. My physical body could not process all the strange foods, bacteria, internal parasites, and other hazards that came with eating unclean foods grown in unclean environments. I became progressively sicker, unable to process any meats or lactose. Fraught with intestinal problems, I came home.

I went to massage school and became a licensed massage therapist. During this time I met and married the man of my dreams. Since then we have had two beautiful children, allowing me to fulfill my greatest desire in life, which was to be a mother. Now I am reliving my childhood through my two children. Nothing could be better than the life I have now.

MY PERFECT WORLD...SHATTERED

But my life wasn't always joyful. My heart has been shattered several times—totally, horridly shattered. The greatest of these heartbreaks came in 2011, two short months after the birth of my son. I lost my best friend, my sister. She made the impulsive decision to end her life the day after her boyfriend was killed in an automobile accident. She left without saying good-bye. I imagine she felt as devastated to lose him as we felt losing her.

Dinah is gone, but she is still everywhere. Still today I can sometimes smell her. I still hear her laugh and see her gestures, the way she used to play with her hair. Sometimes I can almost hear her talking to me. I close my eyes and can feel her around me. I still miss her—terribly. I miss everything about her. Even her imperfections were beautiful. She was spirited. She was creative. She was luminous. She was Dinah, my sister who loved voraciously.

Let me give you one glimpse into the relationship we had. When I was twenty-four or twenty-five years old, I bought a motorcycle. My brother already had one, so he taught me to ride and helped me purchase my first bike. Shortly after, my dad bought one. Then my mom bought one. Then my sister bought one. We all had motorcycles, and a short era of riding together began.

Those times spent with my family were some of the best of my life. We rode everywhere and nowhere. The five of us in our little family bike gang couldn't be stopped.

With Dinah riding beside me, my life was always exciting. One day we traded in our real motorcycles for the Vespa scooter my dad had bought before he had the courage to get a Harley. I drove; she rode on back. We went through the woods and pretended we were Jim Carrey and Jeff Daniels from *Dumb and Dumber*, her favorite movie.

As we were riding around, laughing hysterically at I don't even know what, we saw a pretty large hill with a drop off at the end. Dinah said, "Let's ramp that." I smiled and turned the bike around to gain some speed and distance. We started to pick up speed—fifteen miles per hour, twenty miles per hour, thirty miles per hour, thirty-five miles per hour—and we hit the hill. We gained some serious air, and we were giggling and screaming the whole time like kids on a roller coaster.

We didn't even think about how this scooter would take a landing. It was while we were in the air that I realized the Vespa was not going to land on its tires. We were turning, and as we neared the ground I remember saying to Dinah, "We're gonna crash. Hang on to me."

Instead of her landing on me, I landed on her, and as always she was the injured one and I walked away with only scratches. She banged up her legs and elbows pretty good but didn't require stitches this time.

We still laughed about that incident until the day she died. It was a pure "Jackie and Dinah" moment. It was crazy and impulsive. It was stupid and fun. It was exactly how Dinah and I enjoyed spending our time together. You would think we were teenagers at the time, but we were both grown, married adults!

Memories like these now haunt me yet bring a smile to my face. Somehow, despite her death, Dinah still makes me laugh my face off and cry until my eyes hurt as I remember the crazy times we had together. She was, and still is, the only person who could ever do this to me.

There were other shattering moments, including the loss of three of my children through miscarriage. It wasn't until just recently that I was finally diagnosed with the MTHFR (methylenetetrahydrofolate reductase) genetic mutation. There are several problems associated with the MTHFR gene mutation, but the one that most affected me was miscarriages.

After tears and frustration, my husband and I have decided to be content with our two delightful and precious children. Little Farm Girl is eight years old and is quickly becoming my greatest friend. She is sensitive to my emotions and always wants to please me. Little Farm Boy is six years old. He was born during the most difficult time of my life, but we are now feeling a breath of fresh air—renewal, promise, and the ability to *create joy within our lives*.

I couldn't be happier. Will I always want another child? Probably. Have we thought about adoption? Absolutely. But I want to learn to be satisfied with the life I am living right now and the two living blessings who need all of me.

JOURNEY BACK TO NATURAL

It has been nearly eleven years since I started taking increasingly bigger baby steps toward a more natural, healthy lifestyle. You will read more about this journey in the pages that follow. I have overcome my disease-riddled state and the digestive problems that attacked me in Thailand. I choose now to eat only the foods that are healthy for me. I've struggled with weight issues for years, but I am reaching the point where I understand I must be happy with being the best I can be instead of trying to emulate one of the fake beauty symbols the world throws at me.

> It has been nearly eleven years since I started taking increasingly bigger baby steps toward a more natural, healthy lifestyle.

My husband and I took baby steps to achieve our dream of living on land where we could homestead and produce much of our own food by gardening and raising heritage breed animals. In 2015 we were able to ditch the city and buy our dream farm, where we have ten and a half acres to homestead to our hearts' delight. I still snicker when I look down and see rubber boots instead of polished, tanned toes that complement my one-dollar Old Navy flip-flops.

So today, picnic basket in one hand, my son's hand in the other, I open the rusty gate and head out to find a perfect spot to lay our blanket. The autumn leaves crunch beneath my farm boots. Farm Girl runs ahead of us and asks to let the chickens out. Her wavy hair dances in the mountain air, and she sings a song as the sun flickers off her fading summer highlights. Farm Boy giggles when the chickens break free from their coop, their eyes eager to find juicy bugs outside the coop walls.

Farm Girl picks up her favorite chicken, Susie Sunshine, delicately and gently. This is the second Susie Sunshine. The first met her unfortunate fate when Farm Girl accidentally stepped on her. I felt the blow with her. We held Susie Sunshine's fading body as she slipped away from this world. This was our first hard lesson of farm life, but we knew the pain of death already. I remember when my heart felt crushed, stepped on, like the first Susie Sunshine.

My son slips his hand from mine and brings me back to this moment. I watch as he runs ahead, and I know where he is going. He is fascinated with the "wish flowers" that cover our pasture. He counts to three and blows, and I watch as the white florets surround him and his eyes follow them up in the air above him. The moment is perfect, and I thank God that I am here in it.

At one time, after enduring more loss than I thought my heart could take, I felt like my life was fading away. I couldn't breathe. I was broken and I couldn't hold my head up. My spirit barely was holding on, and I could not get past the pain I felt, body and soul. But as I cried out for help, I felt someone pick me up, and over time God began to ever-so-carefully put me back together.

He gathered all the pieces and put them back in place. He told me, "Gather up the scattered dreams and create the life you love." That is why we named our farm Gather Heritage Farm. It's a place of renewal, restoration, and peace.

I hit my knees on the grass and a wave of peace comes over me. I pull the checkered blanket from our picnic basket, and we sit down to enjoy this day God has given us. My daughter says a prayer and thanks the Lord for her chicken. My son throws his little arms in the air and screams, "Amen!" We break bread together as a little family, one that has been through a few tough years but has come out of the storm.

I had a feeling this place would help me continue to heal, and I'm thankful that it has held up to that expectation. My heart has always longed for more than what a city could offer me—living in it was like a prison.

I'm thankful to be set free.

I'm blessed to be able to treasure this moment. Because now I know how fast life goes by and how quickly things change. Now I know that I can be broken…and happy…and it's OK.

The crushed and broken city girl is gone. A vibrant and peaceful farm girl has arrived.

I'm living a life I once only dreamed, a life that at one time I would never have believed possible. If your dream is to break free of the clutter, reclaim your health, and live simply and close to nature, believe that it is possible. Our family is proof. All you have to do is take one baby step after another, as I did. So let your next step be to keep reading and find out exactly what it means to live an everyday natural life.

Chapter 2

LIVING AN EVERYDAY NATURAL LIFE

*A*RE YOU WONDERING what a natural life really is? There are hundreds of different opinions out there about what natural living is. The entire concept of natural living is constantly evolving. What you learned yesterday, or will learn today, will probably be quite different from what the experts will be saying tomorrow. So let me give you my simple working definition of what natural living is for me and my family.

I will begin by telling you what natural living isn't. It isn't becoming consumed with the need to *do* and *be* everything every expert tells you is part of natural living. It isn't feeling guilty because you can't live up to whoever your perfect idea of "Mrs. Natural" is. It isn't burning the midnight oil boning up on everything written about the natural lifestyle.

Natural living is providing the cleanest, healthiest food, herbal remedies, and household products for my family, avoiding as many chemicals and additives as possible. It is helping each family member to become less stressed, happier, and freer by living as simply and as close to nature as possible.

Natural living isn't transforming into an anxious mess now that you know about all those chemicals, toxins, and GMOs attacking you through commercial foods and products. Before you realized you were choosing harmful ingredients or products that could blow up your health, you were happy. You were oblivious to the dangers in foods and products, and you were enjoying your life. It was nice. Now that you have a little knowledge, you see all these warning labels and artificial food colorings, and you feel like your brain is about to explode. You are constantly afraid you won't be able to keep your family safe from the big, ugly monster called disease that seeks to rob them of their health.

Natural living isn't feeling more stressed, less happy, less functional, and miserable, exhausted, and anxious. It doesn't mean you don't enjoy this beautiful life anymore because you are so overwhelmed by the ugliness in this world. If you no longer enjoy learning about natural and healthy living, if you stress out when new studies come out and feel they put more pressure on you, you're not experiencing the joy of natural living. If you think you *cannot* read another natural living blog or website—if you've blocked them from your feed because you are on healthy education overload and are about to throw in the crunchy natural living towel for good—you definitely are not living the natural lifestyle.

> Natural living isn't feeling more stressed, less happy, less functional, and miserable, exhausted, and anxious.

HOW TO GET STARTED No one wants to feel like that. Natural living is a journey, not a destination, and the most important step you can take is the first one. And it doesn't even have to be a big one. Natural living is taking baby step after baby step. The key is that you are *trying*. You are learning. You are making your home the safest place you can make it for your children.

Just like a little one who is learning to walk, when you take baby steps, sometimes you will fall down. There will be days when you will forget to give your kids their supplements, sneak in a disposable diaper instead of a cloth one, or order that delicious pizza for your family. That's OK. Your family will survive. It isn't the occasional indulgence that hurts us; it's a lifetime of poor choices that eventually brings bad health.

So choose right now to stop trying to live up to your fantasy Pinterest pages and determine to just go back to the basics. Take a moment right now and decide what the five most important steps toward natural living would be for you and your family. Is it adopting a healthier, more organic diet? Is it learning how to make some of your own household products? Maybe it's getting your family to slow down from all their frantic extracurricular activities and spending unscheduled time together. Maybe it's taking time to enjoy the beauty of nature.

What do your children wish for from you? More time? More affection? More togetherness? How about your loved ones and your friends? Do they really want more *things* from you, or do they just want *more of you?*

God's grace covers our guilt and inadequacies and fills us up with joy. So decide today to do the best you can and then leave the rest to God. Tomorrow is a new day, my friends. What baby step will you take then?

For the remainder of this chapter I will give you an overview of some of the first steps many people take as they transition to a natural lifestyle. Everyone who is living a natural lifestyle today started somewhere, and they didn't do everything perfectly fresh out of the gate. They too took a lot of baby steps—and had a lot of falls—before they got it right.

Take Control of the Foods You Eat

A great first step into a more natural lifestyle is determining that you will lead your family into a healthier, less chemical-laden diet. That is a broad topic, and we will take it apart further in later chapters. Here I just want to present some of your options for gradually cleaning up your diet and ridding your life forever of the really nasty chemicals and preservatives you find in over-the-counter food supplies.

Buy organic food options

The word *organic* is the term used to indicate the way fruit, vegetables, grains, and dairy products are grown and processed. Organic farmers use natural, non-chemical fertilizers to nourish the soil and plants, and natural means such as crop rotation or mulch to limit weed growth. There are many reasons people choose organic food. Most are concerned with avoiding the following three things:[1]

+ *Pesticides*—Pesticides are used by conventional growers as a way to prevent mold, disease, and insects from destroying their crops. The residue of these pesticides remains on the harvested produce. Organic farmers do not use harsh chemicals to control pests. Instead they use insect traps, predator insects, or beneficial microorganisms and carefully select disease-resistant crops.

+ *Food additives*—Regulations governing the use of the term *organic* completely restrict growers from using food additives, aids used to process the food but not added directly to the item, and fortifying agents such as "colorings and flavorings," preservatives, artificial sweeteners, and monosodium glutamate (MSG).

+ *Environmental degradation*—Some people buy organic food because of their interest in environmental issues. Organic farming practices reduce pollution and conserve water and soil quality, thus benefitting the environment.

Purchase free-range, grass-fed meats and poultry

When you buy conventional meat and poultry from a grocery store, you can usually tell that some kind of meat lies beneath the plastic wrapping. The label will even tell you what cut of meat you are buying. But those labels *will not* tell you if residues of the rBGH or rBST growth hormones are present or whether trace amounts of the 30 million pounds of antibiotics annually used on livestock can be found in the item.[2] It won't tell you where your meat comes from, how the animals were treated prior to slaughter, or what that animal was fed.

Some grocers are offering organic, grass-fed meats and poultry. But if you want to be sure where your meat comes from, what the animal was fed, and how it was treated, the safest thing to do is to buy directly from a farmer and avoid the grocery store meats and poultry for the most part. We will look closer at how to do this in a later chapter.

Shop at farmer's markets, CSAs, and/or food co-ops

Farmer's markets, community agriculture programs, and co-ops can be great sources for purchasing organic and pesticide-free fruits and vegetables and free-range, grass-fed meats. However, be aware that every farmer's market and co-op is not the same, so you will need to ensure that the produce being sold is organic and pesticide-free, and that the meats actually come from free-range, grass-fed farms. There are some differences between CSAs, farmer's markets, and co-ops, so let me explain what each is:

✦ CSAs (community supported agriculture programs) offer
a direct link between local farmers and consumers. These
CSAs are usually open every week during summer and
fall. Local farmers offer great-tasting, healthy food to their
local CSAs. You can find a variety of vegetables, fruits,
and herbs in season. Some even have milk, farm products, eggs, meat, baked goods, and firewood.[3] CSAs aren't
just good for you and your family; they help to develop
regional food supplies and build strong local economies.

✦ Farmer's markets, farm stands, and "pick-your-own" farms
have become increasingly popular. As I mentioned, not all
farmer's markets sell organic, pesticide-free, and free-range
products, so you will want to do your homework. You can
find a listing of farmer's markets in all fifty states in the
Eat Well Guide (www.eatwellguide.org).

Farm stands are simple roadside tables offering the
products local farms have to offer. But be careful at large
farm stands; they don't always offer *just* local goods.

Pick-your-own farms allow consumers to pick their
own produce (especially berries and fruit) for a set price.
This is really useful for individuals who want to freeze or can a quantity for future use.

> Keep in mind that the best way to find truly grass-fed beef and free-range, organic poultry is to know the farmer.

✦ Food co-ops are groups of people who get together for each member's mutual benefit to purchase sustainable, local, and
organic products. Generally they are volunteer organiza-
tions that don't exist to make a profit, and the only owners
are the members of the co-op. You can check the Co-op
Directory Service to find a co-op in your area.[4]

Whether you purchase food products from a farmer's market,
co-op, or CSA, please keep in mind that the best way to know
whether you are truly buying grass-fed beef and free-range, organic
poultry is to *know the farmer*. Ask questions about his or her
farming practices.

Grow some of your own food

More and more people are taking food production into their own hands—literally—and growing some of their own food. Some people think you need a green thumb to make a garden grow, but with patience, anyone can succeed at gardening.

There are several ways to garden these days.

> ### TIPS FOR PLANTING YOUR OWN GARDEN
>
> If you are fortunate to have some dirt—even a small area—where you can plant vegetables outside, remember these four important tips as you begin:
>
> 1. Don't bite off more than you can chew by planting your garden without considering the time and effort needed to maintain it.
> 2. Be sure you understand the light, soil, water, and nutrient requirements for the vegetables you are planting.
> 3. Know the right time to plant. (See the US Department of Agriculture's Hardiness Zone Map to learn which plants will thrive in your area.)
> 4. Be sure you know how to take care of your plants from planting until harvest.

Container gardening

If you are stuck in an urban area where you see more concrete than dirt when you look out your window, you may want to bone up on container gardening.* You can use just about any container—Smart Pots*; wood, terracotta, or clay pots; an old sink; a wheelbarrow; a rubber boot; a watering trough; or even cardboard boxes or bags of dirt. If you don't have even a small balcony or patio where you can place your containers, consider windowsill gardening from inside your home.

Hydroponic gardening

Hydroponics comes from two Greek words: *hydro* ("water") and *ponics* ("labor"). It refers to soilless gardening, and variations of it have been around for thousands of years. Two early examples of hydroponics are the floating gardens of China and the hanging gardens of Babylon.[5] Many people today are experimenting with their own hydroponic gardens. If this is something you would like to try, you can learn how to build a hydroponic garden at wikihow.com.[6]

You can grow almost any houseplant, fruit, or vegetable you want. Plants with shallow roots are best. As a general rule, hydroponic plants grow faster than traditional garden plants and give higher yields. Many say the flavor and nutrition of hydroponically grown produce exceeds that of soil-grown crops.

Raise some of your own meats and poultry

Some people who are concerned with feeding their families the healthiest foods available have opted to raise some of it themselves. A natural first step into raising meats and poultry is to keep a few of your own chickens. By doing so, you can ensure that your chickens are being raised according to the best organic practices, and you will have a ready supply of roasted or fried chicken and healthy, inexpensive free-range eggs for all your cooking and baking needs. When you are considering this option, just remember these things:

+ Chickens must be fed and watered daily, so if you travel frequently, raising chickens may not be your best option.

+ A freshly roasted chicken sitting on your table is a beauty to behold, but they don't just magically appear there. You will have to butcher the chicken, which can be traumatic for some people.

+ Chickens, like other animals, can be costly to keep. You will need to prepare financially for the expenses of purchasing a flock, and housing and feeding it.

Our own Gather Heritage Farm began with a few chickens. Raising chickens led us to becoming true homesteaders, and we now have ducks, geese, turkeys, rabbits, bees, goats, cattle, sheep, and pigs in our homesteading barnyard. We love our animal family, but we also have committed the time and money it takes to keep them happy, healthy, and safe.

This leads me to the next step you can take toward living an everyday natural lifestyle.

BECOME A RURAL HOMESTEADER

We have met so many people who dream of homesteading someday, but often they don't know how to make that dream a reality. We began our homesteading adventure by renting a farm with only

three acres. It was a perfect start for us, and we were able to successfully explore our farming dreams while saving up to purchase our
dream farm. We began small, which allowed us to gain the experience we needed to purchase and manage our Gather Heritage Farm.

Becoming a homesteader takes careful planning. If this is your
dream, be sure you are setting realistic goals for yourself. The following list may help you determine whether homesteading is right
for you, and help you get started.

1. **Know yourself.** Are you really cut out to be a homesteader? Homesteading is a labor of love involving long
   hours of physical labor for the sheer joy of being able to
   provide for your own needs. Are you up for the challenge?

2. **Set small, achievable goals.** If you're confident that
   you're willing to put in long hours of manual labor, determine your priorities for homesteading. Do you want to be
   totally self-sufficient or just grow your own vegetables in
   your first year?

3. **Make a list** of the tasks you need to complete or things
   you need to have to begin homesteading. Once you've
   made your list, choose five things to accomplish in the
   next six months.

4. **Take inventory of your family.** Is your spouse committed
   to doing this with you? Homesteading takes a commit-
   ment from everyone.

The only way to make your dream of homesteading a reality is
to *get out there and do it*! Do whatever you can to gain the experience and know-how you need. There are tons of resources on homesteading and dozens of homesteaders who will be willing to talk to
you and help you get started. Remember, all homesteaders were new
at one point. We all had to start from ground zero and plan the
work and work the plan to earn the coveted title of *homesteader*.

Frank and I couldn't be happier with our decision to ditch the
city and start a farm. Our kids absolutely adore their new life. They
miss our family in Florida, since our farm is in North Carolina, but
the four of us are our own family, and it's important to my husband
and me to do what's best for our children. The city was scaring me

more and more, and the thought of raising my kids there just kept me up at night. Now they are able to cherish simple things like the joy of collecting eggs, planting seeds and watching them grow, and seeing animals give birth! It's amazing to see how they thrive in this environment.

Success is possible. You just have to tackle homesteading one chicken at a time, one homegrown vegetable at a time, one homemade chicken coop at a time.

> Tackle homesteading one chicken at a time, one homegrown vegetable at a time, one homemade chicken coop at a time.

Whether you choose to homestead, grow a garden, or simply buy organic locally at a grocery store or farmer's market, you will never be sorry. No matter what it looks like for you, taking the first step to living an everyday natural life is so worth it.

PART I

Everyday Natural Food

Chapter 3

EATING REAL FOOD

MY JOURNEY TO a more natural diet simply began with an urgent need to get healthy again. During the year I lived in Thailand, I gradually developed worsening digestive problems from the unhealthy diet I developed there.

Upon my return home to the United States, I began to do some research into the kinds of foods that would make me healthy again. Bit by bit I made wiser choices about my food intake, and with each nutritious, natural food I chose to eat, my health began to return to me. My quest for a healthy, natural diet continued to progress but took years to develop into what it is now.

By the time I had married and had two small children, I was dedicated to a real-food way of eating. For my family, that means eating food that is wholesome and nourishing. It means eating food that is as unchanged by the food industry or by agricultural choices as possible, food that is pure and grown or raised in the most natural ways.

EATING THE *REAL-FOOD* WAY

Moving toward a healthier diet is something many people are trying to do these days. There are dozens of dietary theories and plans people follow. You can take your pick from vegetarian to low-fat to low-carb, blood type, raw, Paleo, and a myriad of other diets. I'll talk more about some of those eating plans later.

If your goal for eating healthier is to lose weight, there are also dozens of weight-loss plans. Some of the most popular include Weight Watchers, Nutrisystem, Jenny Craig, Atkins, and The Biggest Loser. Like many others, I tried many of these diet plans over the years to help me lose weight. Some worked, some didn't, but none led to a continued plan of healthy eating or helped me become more aware of not only the food I put in my mouth but also the chemicals and poisons in those foods.

The more research I did, and the more I talked with others about the dangers existing in processed foods, the more I wanted to learn how to be sure I was eating real food. But what truly constitutes real food? Even though I knew eating real food was what I wanted for myself and my family, I had a lot of questions. I wanted to know:

+ How to start
+ How on earth to make sense of food labels so I could eliminate the bad stuff and still accept the good stuff
+ Whether I could trust my grocery store to provide me with safe, real food
+ Whether our tight family budget could handle the cost of eating better foods, which always seemed to cost more
+ How much additional food preparation time eating real food was going to require since my schedule was already crammed with raising children, attempting to start my own business, and keeping up with household demands

However, once I committed to eating real food, I was determined to understand what real food really was. I couldn't find an official definition of *real food* anywhere, but I was able to develop my own working definition. Real food is not complicated. It's food the way our Creator made it. I wanted to eat single-ingredient food that came straight from the source. And I wanted to know that source so I could be sure it was as pure and natural as advertised.

> Eating real food for our family means eating food that is wholesome, nourishing, and grown or raised in the most natural ways.

I wanted the food we ate to be unprocessed. If any preparation was to be done, I wanted to do it. So I learned about culturing, fermenting, canning, preserving, soaking, and sprouting. As blogger Courtney Dunkin wrote, "Choosing real food is all about avoiding modern agricultural and manufacturing processes and instead going back to the basics."[1]

If these are some of the same choices you want to make for your family, here are a few tips to help you get started.

How to Eat the Real-Food Way

Here are a few simple strategies that can help you begin your journey toward eating real food as a lifestyle.

1. *Change the direction you push your grocery cart in your local food market.* Stop going up and down the aisles, and start circling the perimeter of the store instead. Most of the whole, unprocessed, and unrefined foods in your store can be found around the outside walls.

2. *Don't get trapped by enticing words on food packaging.* Remember, the words on the package are there to make you pick up the food item and buy it. Avoid items with words such as *fortified, enriched, added, extra,* and *plus.* Trust only those items labeled *whole, 100 percent, all natural, certified organically grown, non-GMO,* and *no preservatives.*

3. *Learn to read the small print on food labels.* This puts you in control of what you're eating. Start with the list of ingredients. They are listed in descending order based on how much of that item is in the product. Set a goal to choose single-ingredient foods, but when that is not possible, avoid the products that list damaging items such as sugar and corn syrup as the first ingredients.

4. *Start your own research journey to understand the chemical additives shown in the fine print on food labels.* Sadly these additives may be hidden or barely visible in the list of ingredients. Usually the harder it is to find or read the list of ingredients, the more important it is that you *do* read and understand them. Carry a magnifying glass with you if you

Four Reasons to Shop Local When Possible

- It's usually cheaper.
- It supports the local economy and local farmers.
- It allows you to know about your food.
- It allows you to add your voice to local real food sources.

need to, but take the time to read labels before buying food products. The Healthy Eating Advisor is a great resource to help you understand the items on food labels.[2]

5. *Find a new source for buying your real food.* Shopping the perimeter of your grocery store will help you begin to choose real food, but those foods may not be 100 percent organic or natural and may still contain unsafe additives. Begin finding real-food sources outside the big-box food markets. Start looking for local farmer's markets and get acquainted with farms in your area that offer homegrown produce and raise grass-fed, cage-free, pastured animals.

6. *Find ways to begin growing some of your own foods.* I became so passionate about helping my family eat real food—food that would support a healthier lifestyle and lead us out of the cycle of illness—that I began dreaming of someday growing or raising most of our own food. It was that dream that eventually led us to own our wonderful Gather Heritage Farm.

What is your dream? Do you want to take control of your family's health and know that you are making the healthiest, most nutritious food choices you can make? Then begin *getting in the know!* Take simple steps to eating better. Eat food that is whole, unprocessed, and unrefined.

> Take simple steps to eating better. Eat food that is whole, unprocessed, and unrefined.

Shop at your local farmer's market and choose homegrown, seasonal, organic produce raised without alterations. Look for pasture-raised, grass-fed, and wild poultry, meats, and fish. Eat *real food.*

KEEP IT SIMPLE

When you have decided to fully commit to eating real food, there are some simple steps you can take to move in that direction. Let's look at a few of those.

I've already mentioned that one simple step you can take is to push your grocery cart in a new direction—to stop going up and down the food aisles and start circling the perimeter of the grocery store instead. Most of the real food will be found on the outside walls of the store. So let's use the model of "stop" and "start" to develop some more simple steps.

- STOP using margarine and other substitute butters. START using only real butter.
- STOP using vegetable or canola oils. START using extra-virgin olive oil* (or melted coconut oil*).
- STOP using white and brown sugars. START using stevia,* sucanat,* rapadura,* raw honey, or grade B maple syrup.
- STOP using low-fat or pasteurized, homogenized dairy. START using full-fat dairy (raw if you can find it from trustworthy farms).
- STOP using canned vegetables. START using organic fresh or frozen vegetables.
- STOP using conventional eggs. START using organic, pastured, farm-fresh eggs. (You won't be sorry!)
- STOP using "big agriculture" raised meats. START using organic, grass-fed, pastured meats.
- STOP using farmed fish. START using wild-caught fish.
- STOP using store-bought mayo and salad dressings. START making your own mayo and salad dressings. (Most dressings are made from items you probably already have in your kitchen, such as oil, herbs, and eggs.)
- STOP using store-bought chicken and beef broths. START making your own bone broths.
- STOP using canned soups. START making your own soups.

These few simple substitutions will go a long way toward getting you fully on the path to eating real food every day.

THE TRADITIONAL FOODS MOVEMENT

When I began my journey to eating real food, both my husband and I were dealing with some nagging health issues we wanted to address. Frank seemed unable to bring his cholesterol into a normal range no matter what he did. After two babies in two years, plus the tragic loss of my sister, I carried extra weight and felt miserable physically, mentally, and emotionally.

Through a friend I was introduced to one very healthy eating plan that focused on eating *traditional, real food.* It helps you eliminate foods that are filled with unhealthy additives, preservatives, GMOs, and unhealthy sugars. It consists of eating sustainable meats, poultry, and fish; fresh whole fruits and vegetables; and eggs. This eating plan is how we ensured that we were eating real food. It was the kick-start Frank and I needed to successfully transition to a lifetime of eating real food.

This plan taught me about the importance of eating real, sustainable food and opened me up to a world of slow food (food that is grown, picked, cleaned, and prepared with nutrition in mind—the opposite of fast food) that is nourishing and not threatening to our bodies. The following principles will help you to better understand a traditional foods eating plan:

- The traditional foods eating plan recommends that you cut out all vegetable and hydrogenated oils. This includes all margarines and Crisco, as well as peanut, canola, soybean, and safflower oils. You are encouraged to eat old-fashioned fats in your cooking such as butter from grass-fed cows, lard and bacon fat from pastured pigs, olive oil, and coconut oil.

- It encourages the consumption of sustainable animal protein, including grass-fed red meat, pasture-raised poultry and pork, eggs from truly free-ranging hens, organ meat, wild-caught fish, and shellfish.

- It encourages the consumption of fresh fruits and vegetables that are in season and in flavor! These are enjoyed raw, steamed, cooked, or fermented.

- It advises you to soak rice, grains, beans, and legumes before eating them to deactivate antinutrients.

- It encourages you to eliminate white sugar, sugary drinks, and processed foods and to use healthy sweeteners instead. These include raw, unfiltered honey; unrefined cane sugars such as sucanat or rapadura; molasses; or grade B maple syrup.

+ It encourages you to use full-fat, raw, and fermented dairy.
+ It encourages you to consume eggs only from healthy hens that are truly free-ranging and not contained.

Why not give traditional foods a try? Try it for a month and see how you feel. There are hundreds of traditional-food recipes online and tons of great information to get you started. Choosing traditional foods is one simple, sure way you can feed your family a nutritious, healthy, real-food diet.

But the most important thing is to *just get started*! By doing your own research online you will find dozens of eating plans that can help you take your first steps into eating real food. You can choose one or adopt healthy tips from several as you get started.

The benefits of eating real food are endless. The consequences of not eating real food are tragic. Eating the typical American diet leads to obesity and plays a major role in the development of heart disease, type 2 diabetes, and cancer. You really are what you eat.

When you eat real food, you can know exactly what is going into your body. As one real-food blogger has said:

> The benefits of eating real food go way beyond just your physical health—they help your peace of mind too by giving you the comfort of knowing that you're not filling your body or that of your family with an endless list of ingredients that are full of health risks.[3]

Why don't you begin your own journey to eating real food—*today*? I guarantee that you will be glad you did.

Chapter 4

GROW IT, RAISE IT, OR BUY IT?

WE HAVE BRIEFLY discussed ways to obtain real, nutritious foods. In this chapter I want to take a closer look at the three options of growing your own food, raising your own food, or buying natural, organic food. I will provide some helpful insights regarding each of these options to help you make healthy choices for yourself and your family.

GROWING YOUR OWN FOOD

I'm sure you know by now that I believe growing as many of our own vegetables, fruits, and herbs as possible is the safest way to ensure that we are eating healthy, nutritious, whole foods. But I am just as aware that not everyone has access to the garden plots that will enable them to do so.

I shared some tips in earlier chapters about how to identify safe produce, and I'll give you more later in this chapter. Here I hope to inspire you to realize that you can begin gardening without living on a farm. In fact, if you live in an urban area and don't have a grassy plot, you can grow some simple herbs and vegetables in containers on your concrete patio or in a sunny window in your home. I promise, it's easier than you think.

Plant a container garden

Essentially all you need to plant a container garden is some dirt, something to contain it in, some seeds or starter plants, sunlight, water, and some simple planning. You don't need any special equipment—you can use those old pots and pans you were going to throw out, old compost bags, old wooden buckets, scraps of wood you have lying around, and even things like empty cola bottles. If a container can hold dirt, you can put some drainage holes in the bottom, and it's large enough for your plant's needs, then you can use it for your gardening. Growing a few plants can be done on a very low budget, but you will reap huge benefits in your journey to eating healthy, real food.

You can put your containers on whatever little piece of out-doors you have, but if you have an area inside where natural light flows for at least a few hours each day, it is possible to grow some of your own food indoors too. Try planting your

> If a container can hold dirt, you can put some drainage holes in the bottom, and it's large enough for your plant's needs, then you can use it for your gardening.

own herb garden on a windowsill so you can have fresh basil, rosemary, parsley, chives, and other herbs ready as you need them.

You can also grow vegetables in containers. Miniature forms of larger vegetables such as tomatoes, pumpkins, and squash are well suited to containers. Or you can plant a salad garden filled with colorful lettuces, dwarf tomatoes, chives, peppers, and cucumbers. Space doesn't have to keep you from growing your own food.

Plan a backyard garden plot

A small, manageable backyard garden plot is another great way to grow healthy, organic vegetables, and it will provide wholesome activities and experiences for the entire family. If you have space to plant a garden in your yard, keep the following in mind.

+ Keep your plot at a size you can maintain because you will have to put in the work necessary to keep it growing. But you don't need a huge plot. A simple ten-by-ten-foot plot can give you a steady supply of salad makings for your family.

+ Be sure your plants face south and get a minimum of five hours of sunlight daily.

+ Keep your garden away from the tree drip lines (which are used for irrigation) to avoid their encroaching root systems.

+ Be sure to prepare and enrich your soil before you start. Soil test kits are available from your local county extension office for this purpose and can tell you what you need to enrich your soil.

+ If possible, start a compost bin. This will give you continued nutrients to fuel your plants and restore depleted soil.

TIPS FOR ORGANIC GARDENING[1]

- Plan your garden before planting to reap the best harvest.
- Less is more. Start small and expand each season.
- Choose plants that will grow well in your region's climate and geography.
- Share and barter. Share seeds and seedlings with your friends and neighbors.
- Use organic supplies. There are many natural products that can be used to treat weeds, diseases, pests, and soil issues.
- Give your plants a companion. Do your research and grow plants that benefit one another.
- Have fun! Gardening can be a wonderful bonding experience for the whole family.

+ Use only organic, natural substances for any pest control you need.

Choose easy crops to begin with. The easiest tomatoes to grow are cherry tomatoes, and herbs such as rosemary, thyme, and basil are pretty much foolproof crops. Beans, radishes, green onions, spinach, and leaf lettuces mature quickly, and you can plant them between rows of longer-maturing plants such as tomatoes, peppers, and cabbage. Determine how much you want to harvest of each vegetable crop to meet your family's needs.

The important thing is to just get started. Gardening will ensure that you are providing your family with wonderful, healthy, real food. And taking these first small steps into gardening is a fantastic way to prepare to fulfill your dreams of someday having your own farm. Now, go and get your garden on!

CHOOSING THE SAFEST MEAT

I know that not everyone reading this book can—or even wants to—begin homesteading on a farm of their own. But that doesn't mean you can't be sure you're serving your family safe grass-fed and pastured poultry and meats.

Know the common terms

Not all meats that have been declared safe really are safe. Savvy marketers use creative terminology to get consumers to believe their product is worth purchasing. If your goal is to buy the safest meat possible, you'll want to get familiar with the following terms.

- Grass-fed—The US Department of Agriculture (USDA) defines *grass-fed* as meat from "ruminant" animals such as cattle and sheep that survive on grass. So if you see this term on items such as pork or eggs, buy another brand.

- Free-range—The USDA has a vague definition for free-range poultry, but it may not be what you picture when you think of the term—poultry roaming free on roomy pastures. Some poultry are considered free-range even if they are cooped up most of the time on a barn floor and only occasionally allowed access to a feces-laden concrete pad or pasture.

- Grass-finished—Large-scale farms sometimes ready an entire herd for slaughter all at once by finishing their readiness with grain-based feed. In that short period of time just about all the healthy benefits of eating grass are eliminated.[2] But the term *grass-finished* is not a common term, so it's best to simply ask your beef source farmers.

- American Grassfed Association (AGA) certification—*Organic* and *grass-fed* do not always mean what they say. The AGA certification is the only one that means the animals eat nothing but grass for their entire lives.

It is important that you know your farmer. The best way to be sure you are getting real grass-fed beef is to get to know the farmer growing your food. You should be buying your beef from a farmer who can tell you how he treats his animals and how he gets them ready for slaughter.

Know where to find cage-free, free-range, pastured poultry

Once again the safest way to determine that the poultry and eggs you are purchasing are both organic and truly pasture-raised is to know the farmer or food source providing those items to you. Chickens are raised very differently today than they were in the "old days." Most supermarket chickens never see the light of day and may be only six or seven weeks old when they are sent off to be butchered. They are crammed together with thousands of other birds and often don't have even enough room to spread their wings. Their beaks have been cut off so they won't peck each other to death from the frustration created by their unnaturally close quarters. Now you know why chicken and eggs don't taste like they used to.[3]

It is for these reasons, and because we want to be sure the food we eat is as organic and free of pesticides and chemicals as possible, that we raise both egg-laying hens and meat chickens. But you may not be able to raise your own poultry.

It is important for you to be aware that the labels "cage-free," "free-range," and "pastured" are often little more than creative advertising. Truly free-range or pasture-raised hens forage freely for their food from pastures. These pastures have all they need for their natural diet, which will include seeds, green plants, insects, and worms.

If you have access to them, local farmers who allow their hens to forage freely outdoors are your best source for poultry. If you live in a large city or in an area where there is no ready access to direct source farms, the local health food stores are usually the best way to find high-quality egg sources. Even in large cities you can find farmer's markets where you can get to know the people who grow your food.

Know how to identify truly safe seafood

Fish are your best source of omega-3 fats EPA and DHA. But as Dr. Joseph Mercola notes, with the levels of pollution increasing, we must be very selective about the kinds of seafood we eat. Many fish species are being raised on fish farms where they are fed GMOs, pesticides, antibiotics, and various other chemicals used to combat diseases and parasites in fish.[4]

Make a decision to avoid as much farm-raised seafood as possible. While it may be difficult to determine whether packaged fish was farm-raised or wild-caught, there are some useful ways to choose safe seafood:[5]

+ Look for wild-caught Alaskan and sockeye salmon. These are among the best salmon options because they tend to be safe from contamination and contain the highest amounts of healthy omega-3 fat. Neither is allowed to be farmed.

+ When choosing canned fish, look for smaller fish such as sardines, anchovies, and herring.

+ Watch for the words *fishwise* and *seafood safe* on packaging. The fishwise label identifies how and where the fish was caught, and whether it is sustainable or threatened. The seafood safe label "involves independent testing of fish for contaminants, including mercury and PCBs [polychlorinated biphenyls, a group of manufactured organic chemicals that pollute some water supplies], and recommendations for consumption based upon the findings."[6]

PURCHASING SAFE, REAL FOOD FROM A GROCER

The fact that you are reading this book most likely means you are working to get processed foods out of your diet and provide more real food for your family. For most of us, the great majority of our food will come from the larger grocery stores. In this final section I want to assure you that you can find organic, nutritious, safe, real food at your local grocery store. I want to help you do this by suggesting some things to be aware of as you shop.[7]

Shopping for produce

When you start cooking real food, you will spend a lot of your time in the produce section of your local grocery store. Try to buy as much 100 percent certified organic and locally grown produce as you can afford.

Do some research on what *not* to purchase. You can find

THE DIRTY DOZEN[8]	
1. Strawberries	7. Cherries
2. Spinach	8. Grapes
3. Nectarines	9. Celery
4. Apples	10. Tomatoes
5. Peaches	11. Sweet bell
6. Pears	peppers
	12. Potatoes

a list of the "dirty dozen" produce online. This list, updated annually, names the most pesticide-laden, over-sprayed crops. Be sure you purchase only organic varieties of the produce on this list or, better still, get them from a local farmer's market where the growers can vouch for their safety. Be aware that corn, summer squash, and zucchini are largely genetically modified, so it's worth it to pay the extra cost for organic.

Your budget will probably dictate that you must get some nonorganic items. Research the "clean fifteen" list and focus on purchasing conventional versions of only those items.

Dairy

Purchase full-fat, organic dairy (raw, if possible). If organic dairy is not available, look for dairy from grass-fed cows. Refuse to buy any processed cheeses you see on the shelves. Also avoid any dairy from cows that have been given hormones. If you cannot find hormone-free cheeses, opt for cheeses that still have their natural white color.

If you cannot find hormone-free milk, choose coconut or almond milk. I recommend that you avoid soy milk.

Eggs

Look to buy organic eggs from chickens that are free-range, cage-free, and certified humanely raised. Read the packaging carefully to ensure that your eggs meet all these benchmarks.

THE CLEAN FIFTEEN[9]

1. Sweet corn
2. Avocados
3. Pineapples
4. Cabbage
5. Onions
6. Sweet peas (frozen)
7. Papayas
8. Asparagus
9. Mangos
10. Eggplant
11. Honeydew melon
12. Kiwi
13. Cantaloupe
14. Cauliflower
15. Grapefruit

Meat, poultry, and seafood

I've already given you tips for buying your meats, poultry, and seafood. Follow that advice and do your best to buy organic meat and wild-caught seafood.

Frozen foods

Pass up the premade, processed meals and pre-seasoned frozen veggies, and choose organic frozen produce and meats that have no additives or seasoning.

Condiments

It's best to make your own condiments, but if you must buy them, avoid any that include soy, high-fructose corn syrup, or ingredients that you can't pronounce. Get as many organic versions as possible with less than five added ingredients.

Sweeteners

As I mentioned previously, the better sweeteners are raw, unfiltered honey; unrefined cane sugar; grade B maple syrup; stevia; and blackstrap molasses. Say good-bye to white sugar. Leave behind brown sugar (coconut sugar is a great substitute), Karo syrup, agave nectar (which is highly processed), and other artificial sweeteners.

Baking supplies

Purchase einkorn flour* (an heirloom flour with more protein, vitamin B_6, phosphorous, and potassium than more modern forms of wheat); whole wheat or white whole wheat flour; and coconut, olive, or grapeseed oils. Don't even go down the aisle that contains premade baked goods. Try some recipes that use coconut flour or almond flour instead of wheat flour if you are looking to avoid gluten.

Don't forget that there are many organic, real-food options you can buy online. And start making those weekly trips to your local farmer's markets and farm stands for your real food needs.

Whether you grow your food or buy it from a grocery store or a local farm, you can find good, whole food that will nourish your body and improve your health. If you follow the tips I've shared in this chapter and remember to push your grocery cart around the perimeter of the store and not up and down the aisles, you will find yourself moving toward the goal of transitioning to eating healthy, real food as a lifestyle.

Chapter 5

DEVELOPING YOUR NATURAL EATING PLAN

*H*ERE IN PART 1, I have showed you some "baby steps" you can take to begin a healthier, more natural way of eating. I've given you some basic tips both for shopping for healthier, organic food products and for growing some of your own fruits and vegetables, and possibly even raising some of your own meat and poultry.

In this chapter I want to dig a bit more into some of the specific benefits you can derive from selecting certain natural, organic food products. I want to start with a simple list of some easy substitutions you can make for healthier eating. Each of the substitutions you make from this list will be a big step on your journey to a healthier eating lifestyle.

SIMPLE SUBSTITUTIONS FOR A HEALTHIER MENU

TRADITIONAL INGREDIENT	REAL-FOOD OPTIONS
All-purpose white flour	Whole wheat flour, coconut flour, almond flour
White or brown sugar	Sucanat or coconut sugar, stevia, raw honey, maple syrup
Cornstarch	Arrowroot powder*
Margarine, shortening, or vegetable oil	Real butter or coconut oil, palm shortening, extra-virgin olive oil, ghee

TRADITIONAL INGREDIENT	REAL-FOOD OPTIONS
Table salt	Real sea salt
Store-bought mayo	Homemade mayo with healthy oils
Low-fat, pasteurized, and homogenized dairy products	Full-fat dairy or raw dairy (when you can get it)
Store-bought peanut butter	Almond or cashew butter, homemade or all-natural peanut butter
Store-bought chicken and beef broths	Homemade bone broth
Store-bought salad dressings	Homemade dressings using olive oil and vinegar
Conventionally raised meat	Organic, grass-fed, pastured meat
Conventional eggs	Organic, pastured, farm-fresh eggs
Canned vegetables and fruits	Fresh or frozen vegetables and fruits
Commercial bacon and sausages	Uncured, nitrate-free bacon and sausage
Lunch meat and cold cuts	Thinly sliced home-cooked meats or nitrate-free deli or lunch meats

This chart gives you good options to help you start choosing more natural, healthier food products. As you continue your journey, you will want to develop your personal eating plan even further and will likely want to make some food choices beyond these beginning steps.

For example, there may come a time when you are fully convinced that you and your family could eat healthier by eliminating gluten, and possibly all grains, from your eating plan. At that point your substitutions will be gluten-free or grain-free choices. Or through your personal research you may discover farm stores, co-ops, or online sites where you can purchase the specialty grass-fed, organic, pastured meats you want for your family. But the information I have shared with you thus far will help you train yourself to make healthier choices every time you go to the store to purchase a food item.

SOME OF MY FAVORITE NATURAL-FOOD CHOICES

My husband and I have been developing our own healthy, natural eating style for several years. There are many specific natural, organic choices that we use in our daily eating plans. We have committed to raising only certain heritage breed animals (for both breeding and as food sources) and growing only the natural, organic fruits and vegetables we most want to include in our eating plan. For those food items we do not grow or raise ourselves, we try to shop or trade only at our local farmer's markets, co-ops, or produce stands, where we can get organic, natural products we can trust. For the remainder of our food purchases, we make sure we are buying only organic, natural products from local grocery stores or from our favorite online markets.

We chose some of the items in our eating plan because of their overwhelming health benefits. I want to mention some of those powerhouse natural foods because I highly recommend them to your family also.

Homemade bone broths and stocks

There is a South American proverb that says, "Good broth will resurrect the dead."[1] While that is no doubt an exaggeration, it shows that this food has long been considered a wholesome addition to the human diet. Because of modern meat processing techniques, it is very difficult to find healthy stocks and broths. Even the organic broths often come from beef and poultry raised according to traditional methods, which are generally unhealthy and nutrient-stripping.

When properly prepared, meat and bone stocks are extremely nutritious, as they contain minerals from the bones, marrow, and cartilage along with electrolytes from the vegetables. I've also learned that adding an acidic medium raw apple cider vinegar makes the stock even more nutritious by helping to draw out even more minerals, including magnesium and potassium.

There is magic in homemade stock that cannot be found in the chicken- or beef-flavored water sold in stores. Another advantage of making homemade stock is that it's just so easy. My method for making healthy homemade stock has become second nature and can be done in six easy steps.

Homemade Bone Broth

1. I always plan on eating a whole chicken a week. I rinse the chicken, put the organs in the fridge for the stock, throw the chicken in the slow cooker (breast side down), add two to four cups of water (depending on the size of the bird), and then cook the chicken on low for six to eight hours. I know it's done when the legs easily fall off.

2. I then let the chicken cool. Once it has cooled, I take all the meat off and throw the skin, bones, and organs back into the slow cooker.

3. I cut an onion in fourths and throw it in the slow cooker along with two whole garlic cloves, about an inch-long piece of ginger, one celery stalk, one carrot, half a cup of apple cider vinegar, and a chicken foot (for added gelatin) if I have one.

4. I then fill the rest of the slow cooker with water. I set it to low and let it simmer for twenty-four to forty-eight hours.

5. About an hour before I am ready to turn off the slow cooker, I add my spices: salt, pepper, and sage.

6. I let the broth simmer for one more hour, let it cool, and then strain the stock.

The outcome is amazing! The broth is so dark and beautiful. If you have an Instant Pot pressure cooker, then you can follow the same method, but it will take you only ninety minutes to complete step four! Yes, I get excited about it! When I see bones, I think of all the wonderful stocks I can make with them. I usually plan on making some kind of soup every week. Sometimes I freeze the stock. You can also boil the stock down and put it in ice cube trays. It's so easy and so frugal to make stock.

Raw-milk dairy products

If you have followed my blogging over the years, you will know that my family chooses many of our foods from a Paleo eating plan, which does not normally include grains, sugars, legumes, or dairy. However, I have refused to be locked into a rigid "If you don't do this, you aren't really Paleo" mind-set. While we greatly appreciate the healthy aspects of this way of eating, we make as many other real-food choices outside of the Paleo eating plan as we believe are right for our family. One of the healthy choices we make is drinking raw milk and making dairy products from raw milk.

> When I see bones, I think of all the wonderful stocks I can make with them!

Raw milk is milk that has not been through the pasteurization process. Pasteurization is a heating process that is supposed to kill disease-causing germs and bacteria, but it often destroys the health benefits of the milk as well. Our Gather Heritage Farm includes cattle in our barnyard menagerie. We love the raw milk we get from our milk cow and use it both to drink and to make cheese products. Let me share some good reasons why we drink raw milk.

1. Because we raise our own milk cow, I know the source and quality of our milk. We know exactly what she is eating, and we keep her in our controlled lush, green pastures to graze. In contrast, unless labeled otherwise, you can bet store-bought milk is completely grain-fed—even organic milk.

2. It improves our oral health. Raw milk is very rich in vitamins A, D, K, and B-complex. Moreover, fresh raw milk contains more vitamin C, which is decreased by up to 25 percent through pasteurization.[2] All these vitamins are extremely necessary for good oral health.

3. Raw milk is very high in calcium. Many people have been told that milk makes them sick, or they can't digest dairy or may have experienced negative side effects from drinking pasteurized milk. However, for the majority of these people, these negative effects do not occur when they drink raw milk. However, eliminating raw milk from your diet brings up the question of where to get proper calcium. On average, an adult needs somewhere between 1,000 and 1,200 mg of calcium per day.[3] On a dairy-free diet you will need to consume lots of vegetables, one to two cups of bone broth, and a moderate amount of seafood to get the adequate calcium in your diet.

If you want to get an idea of where your milk comes from, go to a local farm and ask if you can help with milking the cows. The kids will love it! My youngest was recently able to milk a cow and pointed the stream of milk toward his mouth! Yes, he was trying to aim the milk into his mouth. My children have only known good, real, raw milk. They won't drink anything else.

Apple cider vinegar

Most people wouldn't even consider apple cider vinegar (ACV) a staple for their menu plans, but this age-old, healthy product has a surprising number of uses. Because of its beneficial qualities, I believe it is important to consider making ACV a regular addition to your eating plans. Here are just a few of the benefits of ACV:

+ Drinking a tablespoon of ACV in a glass of water before meals can improve digestion and stop tummy troubles such as indigestion, bloating, and heartburn in their tracks.[4]

+ Rinsing your hair with one part ACV and one part water after washing helps to balance its pH level, leaving your hair softer, smoother, and healthier.[5]

+ Mixing a tablespoon of ACV with a teaspoon of honey can greatly alleviate problems caused by having too much acid in the body, including arthritis and gout.[6] ACV's ability to balance the body's pH level can also help reduce the risk of cancer.[7]

+ Drinking a mixture of ACV and water after a workout provides potassium and other nutrients and enzymes that assist with recovery.[8]

+ ACV is often used to help in weight loss and weight management, and it helps support healthy blood glucose and insulin levels.[9]

If you purchase raw, unpasteurized ACV with "the mother" (the beneficial acids and bacteria that make the vinegar look cloudy) and use it regularly, even if just in your homemade salad dressings, you will be taking a wonderful step toward getting the benefits of regular ACV consumption.

Coconut oil

Coconut oil is so healthy for you and your family. It has many benefits, and there are many ways to use it. Natural coconut oil is full of antioxidants and healthy saturated fats, and it contains medium-chain fatty acids that are extremely beneficial to our health.[10] It is one of the healthy oils that I recommend you switch to, leaving behind the unhealthy vegetable, soy, and canola oils you may be accustomed to using.

There are many ways to incorporate healthy coconut oil into your diet.

+ Use it as a cooking oil and add it to your smoothies, sauces, and homemade desserts.

+ Try adding it to your coffee or tea in the morning by blending it thoroughly with an immersion blender.* This is called bulletproof coffee.

+ Use it in your homemade toothpaste and for oil pulling for healthier teeth (see chapter 7 for more on this).

+ Add it to your children's bathwater at night and use it to gently massage your little ones' skin. It prevents many irritating skin problems and leaves their skin soft and smooth as butter.

Be sure to purchase 100 percent virgin coconut oil produced by using a "wet-milling process." This means the oil has been extracted from fresh coconut meat without drying the meat first. It is the best coconut oil for you.

A REAL-FOOD BREAKFAST, LUNCH, AND DINNER

When you are just beginning to make the switch to natural, organic food products and to eliminate the foods with unhealthy chemicals, preservatives, and additives, you may struggle to figure out what specific menu item you want to serve at a certain meal. To help you begin planning healthier menus, let me give you one healthy recipe each for breakfast, lunch, and dinner. These are dishes my family loves to eat over and over again, and they can help to jump-start your own journey to healthier, more natural living.

Healthy sweet potato breakfast cookies

Sweet potatoes are a staple in our kitchen. They are easy to grab, great for helping you recover from a hard workout, and loaded with healthy carbohydrates. They have massive amounts of beta-carotene and contain more fiber than white potatoes. They have high levels of vitamin B_6, manganese, and potassium; are rich in vitamins C and E; and contain iron, magnesium, and vitamin D.[11] I adapted these Sweet Potato Breakfast Cookies from a recipe you can find online from The Preppy Paleo.[12] My family loves these cookies warm from the oven for breakfast or at any time of day when we need a healthy snack. As I write this, I'm eating them for breakfast with some bacon! My kids are devouring them too and think I'm the coolest mom for letting them have cookies for breakfast! Here's a tip: Always make a double recipe. They freeze well too.

Sweet Potato Breakfast Cookies

½ cup almond butter
½ cup pureed sweet potato (roast in the oven or microwave for six minutes)
¼ cup natural maple syrup or raw honey
2 eggs
½ tsp. vanilla
½ tsp. baking soda
1 tsp. cinnamon

½ tsp. nutmeg

½ tsp. real salt (or Himalayan sea salt)

2–3 cups of your choice of mix-ins: coconut shreds, chocolate chips, raisins, almond slivers, walnuts, cranberries, pumpkin seeds, hemp hearts, etc.

Preheat the oven to 350 degrees. Combine all the ingredients in a large bowl. Drop by 1–2 tablespoonfuls onto a greased, parchment paper–lined or silicone baking sheet. Press down slightly with your palm. Bake for 12–15 minutes until golden brown. The recipe should make twelve large breakfast cookies for you to enjoy.

Taco lunch salad with pork or chicken

My family really enjoys a good salad for lunch. We have found that this Green Chile Taco Salad is just the thing to fill us up and energize us for the rest of our busy day on Gather Heritage Farm. I often have leftover pulled pork or pulled chicken from a meal made earlier in the week. To keep this healthy, be sure to use chicken or pork from grass-fed, organic, pastured meats you have purchased from a healthy source.

Green Chile Taco Salad

Approximately 1–2 cups of leftover pulled pork or chicken

1–2 Tbsp. olive oil or coconut oil

1 tsp. ground cumin

1 tsp. garlic powder

1 tsp. sea salt

1 tsp. oregano

1–2 cups green or red enchilada sauce (I recommend El Pato Hot Tomato Sauce)

Garnishes of your choosing: cilantro, olives, cheddar cheese, sour cream, romaine, tomatoes, guacamole or sliced avocado, salsa, and plantain chips

Assuming you are using leftover pulled chicken or pork, put the olive or coconut oil in a large sauté pan and add the chicken or pork, spices, and enchilada sauce. Heat to medium hot and simmer for 10 minutes to merge the spices and sauce with the meat. Place the slightly cooled meat mixture on a bed of romaine lettuce and garnish with the foods of your choice. This makes a delicious lunchtime salad.

Beef stroganoff dinner

This dish is so good, I just can't keep it to myself anymore! I make it two to three times a month. It's just so delicious and comforting. It is nourishing and 100 percent grain-free! You can also make it dairy-free by using coconut milk cream instead of sour cream. I hope you like it!

Ground Beef Stroganoff

2 Tbsp. butter or ghee
2 Tbsp. olive oil or coconut oil, divided
1 large onion, chopped
8 oz. sliced white mushrooms
1 lb. ground beef
2 Tbsp. tomato paste
1½ tsp. dried thyme
1½ tsp. dried rosemary
4 cloves garlic, minced
1 Tbsp. arrowroot powder
1½ cups beef stock (or use your homemade chicken or beef broth)
⅔ cup thick coconut cream
½ tsp. sea salt
½ tsp. black pepper
Cooked cauliflower rice, spiralized zucchini "noodles," or spaghetti squash

Melt the butter or ghee with 1 tablespoon olive or coconut oil over medium heat. Add onions and mushrooms and sauté until slightly softened and browned. Remove to a plate. Brown the ground beef in 1 tablespoon olive oil until no longer pink. Return onions and mushrooms to the pan. Mix in the tomato paste, thyme, rosemary, and garlic, and sauté for about 3 minutes to develop the flavors.

Reduce to medium heat. Sprinkle arrowroot powder over the mixture and stir until thoroughly combined. Stir in beef stock and fully incorporate. The sauce will thicken as it comes to a simmer. Reduce heat and simmer for 5 minutes. Remove pan from heat and let mixture cool for a couple of minutes. Stir in the sour cream or coconut cream. Serve over your choice of cauliflower rice, zucchini noodles, or roasted spaghetti squash.

Serves 6–10 people.

I believe this chapter has given you the tools you need to begin your own journey to healthy meal planning. Now it's your turn. Take your first steps and try my suggestions. If you do, I'm confident your appetite will be begging for more healthy food options. Eating natural, healthy meals is such a powerfully enjoyable and beneficial way of life. I know you are going to love it.

PART II

Everyday Natural Body

Chapter 6

DEALING WITH
ISSUES OF WEIGHT

OR MANY PEOPLE, body weight is the proverbial elephant that is always in the room. We are constantly bombarded with images of women shaped like Barbie dolls and given the subtle message over and over again that if you are too thin or too fat, you are just not good enough. The problem with this thinking is that it leads people to have a negative body image and to constantly compare their bodies to others'. It leads them to feel shame, anxiety, and self-consciousness about their appearance. A poor body image can lead to all sorts of negative feelings, including low self-esteem, depression, unhappiness, and obsession with weight loss. It can even lead to an eating disorder.

The cause of this weight and body image epidemic is the way we eat. In our busy lives too often we choose convenience over health. There are fast-food restaurants all over, and it's so much easier to go through a drive-through for a burger and fries for lunch than to prepare a healthy, real-food lunch. It's so much easier to pick up a few prepackaged freezer meals for dinner or to eat out and consume a big meal loaded with extra calories than to come home after a long day of work and face the chore of cooking the evening meal.

The problem is that fast-food meals and prepared dinner entrees are loaded with extra sugars, fats, and unhealthy additives and chemicals. One recent food chart shows that processed food makes up 63 percent of the calories we eat daily.[1] Sadly plant-based *real food* makes up only 12 percent of the calories consumed in the United States.[2] Unfortunately the standard American diet (SAD) has had a devastating effect on many Americans. It has led to epidemic levels of obesity, which is contributing to a sharp rise in hypertension, heart disease, and diabetes.[3]

Like many Americans, I battled my own war with weight for years. I was suckered into wanting to look like the models on TV and felt inadequate or less than OK because I just could not get there, or if I did get there, I couldn't seem to stay there. In this chapter I want to help you find ways to kick that weight elephant right out of the room. I want to focus on two main things:

+ Making the right food choices to achieve a healthy weight
+ Developing a better body image

It seems almost too easy to say, "Wrong foods = weight gain; right foods = weight loss," but that is often exactly the way it happens. But bringing your weight into a healthier range will not fully change your body image. Some of those changes have to take place in your mind and spirit. Let's get started.

MAKING HEALTHY FOOD CHOICES

I am certainly an example of the "wrong foods = weight gain; right foods = weight loss" mantra. Wrapped up in that is the fact that weight issues led me to develop a poor body image and caused lingering health problems that needed to improve. My eating habits in Thailand were those of convenience. It was much easier to just pick up street food every day than to find the ingredients to make food that would be healthy for me. Many of the grocery items I could find, though appropriate for healthy salads and meals, were really unclean and unhealthy because of the way they were grown and sold. Produce grew in unsafe soil and water conditions, and meats and poultry hung in open-air markets where they picked up all forms of bacteria. Not only did I gain weight, I also gained bad health.

Unfortunately, the standard American diet (SAD) has led to epidemic levels of obesity, hypertension, heart disease, and diabetes.

Back in the United States, once I had suffered through several months of getting my health back, I picked right back up with the standard American diet. Young and single, I found it so much easier to get fast, convenient food than to learn to buy and prepare real food.

Somewhere along the way I did become more sensitized to the need to make better food choices, and I gradually moved to a real-food diet. But because my body image still had not changed, when stress, pregnancies, and loss hit me, I fell back into making food choices based on my negative emotions, choosing comfort foods such as greasy hamburgers, baked goods, pizza, and bulky carbohydrates. I knew I needed a change, and I needed it *now*! I needed to learn how and what to eat.

Discovering the traditional and real-food way of eating became the tool that helped me get rid of the weight elephant once and for all. But hear me on this: I wasn't just able to shed some pounds; just as important was the fact that I learned to develop a better body image, one not based on weight alone but on feeling good about myself for reasons other than just my weight. I learned to express my positive feelings through family activities, fun adventures, and great relationships.

Here I want to show you some ways to move from unhealthy food choices to eating naturally with real food. No one plan is the answer; it is a matter of simply learning to make the right food choices consistently. A healthy body and body image begins with eating real food.

Remember what real food is? As one health blogger wrote, real food is "things that grew in the ground, on a tree, came out of the sea, ran on the land, or flew through the air. Meat, fish, eggs, vegetables, fruits, [and] nuts are all great examples of REAL food."[4]

It will be very important for you to remember as you begin to make real food choices that you cannot simply *add* these items to your current menu. Unless you begin to *subtract* your junk-food choices, you will not be successful at either losing weight or changing your body image.

But bear in mind that if you are changing your eating habits because you think you should, you will soon falter. It's not easy to give up those favorite comfort foods. The only way to succeed is to keep focused on your goal—a healthier, natural life. That goal is not out of your reach, but you must commit to making a change.

HOW TO TRANSITION TO BETTER FOOD CHOICES

Losing weight is all about the food, and how much of it, you choose to eat. For most of us, learning to eat real food is a matter of exchanging an unhealthy food for a healthy one. It will be different for each person, but in this section I want to look at the food groups and some healthy substitutions you can make to begin a weight-loss journey.

Keep in mind that these are baby steps. You may not be able to transition to a completely natural diet all at once. For that reason, there are some options given

> You must make a commitment to change.

that are not entirely natural and that you eventually may want to remove from your diet completely. Even if these are not all ideal options, they are better choices that will get you moving in a healthier direction. When you are starting your journey to natural living, your first baby steps may not be fully natural, as these recommendations will show, but they will get you moving in the right direction.[5]

Grains

Choose whole-grain breads and bakery items over foods made with white flour. They are lower in fat and higher in fiber and complex carbs, which help you to feel fuller longer. When choosing grains, look at the list of ingredients on the packages and choose the ones that have the word *whole* in front of the grain or flour. Instead of sugary cereals and regular granolas, choose oatmeal and whole-grain cereal. Stay away from rich bakery treats and fried snacks such as potato chips. Try unsalted whole-grain pretzels and homemade popcorn instead (never use microwave popcorn, which is very unhealthy). Choose whole-wheat pasta and brown rice over white rice.

Fruits and vegetables

Fresh fruits and vegetables are naturally low in fat; what gets many of us in trouble is adding sugary syrups and butter or margarine, mayo, and sour cream. Instead of fried vegetables served with cream, butter, or cheese sauces, choose to steam, broil, or bake raw vegetables and toss them with a small amount of olive oil and salt and pepper. Leave the french fries behind for a tasty baked white or sweet potato.

Meat, poultry, and fish

Try to buy organic meats, or meat from a local farmer. (See the appendix for resources to help you find local sources of organic meat in your area.) If you cannot find these meats or it isn't in your budget, then choose lean cuts and trim the outside fat before cooking. (Grass-fed meats typically have less fat overall and a higher concentration of the good omega-3 fats.[6]) Season meats with herbs, spices, fresh veggies, and organic marinades, but avoid high-sugar sauces and gravies.

Baking, broiling, roasting, and grilling are the healthiest ways to prepare meat and poultry. The healthiest ways to prepare fish and seafood, which you should try to eat twice a week, are poaching, steaming, baking, and broiling. Instead of buying breaded fish items or fish canned in canola oil, choose fresh or frozen fish and canned fish in water.

Avoid processed lunch meats as much as possible. If you do eat processed lunch meats, choose ones that are labeled as "nitrate-free."

Dairy

Substitute heavy whipping cream for sugar-laden coffee creamers. You won't be sorry! (In time you may even want to try adding coconut oil to your coffee, as I do with my bulletproof coffee.) Try whole-milk cheeses and milk over low-fat cheese or skim milk. Choose whole-milk yogurt instead of low-fat. This may seem unconventional, but studies have found that when people eat less fat they tend to consume more sugar, which contributes to weight gain.[7]

Fats, oils, and sweets

Avoid foods and oils filled with too much saturated and trans fat. Instead of sugar-sweetened drinks such as fruit juice, regular soft drinks, sports drinks, energy drinks, and sweetened tea, choose water, zero-calorie flavored water (infused water is worth a try, as you'll want to avoid artificial sweeteners), and unsweetened tea. Instead of cookies or potato chips for snacks, choose a piece of fresh fruit with a small piece of cheese, plain yogurt mixed with fruit, or fresh veggies dipped in savory flavored yogurt.

WEIGHT LOSS REQUIRES MORE THAN A DIET

There are hundreds of diet plans available, and like me, you've probably tried a great many of them. But successfully losing weight requires much more than simply following a rigid diet plan for a specified period of time. Being truly successful at taking weight off and keeping it off requires lifestyle changes that revolutionize not only your eating habits but also the entire way you live your life.

Many times you just need to make some simple, small adjustments. Perhaps you stop eating lunch out at some fast-food restaurant and start taking healthy, wholesome lunches to work with you. Or instead of parking as close to the store as you can get, you park farther away and walk a few hundred feet instead. It's important that you change your perspective. New habits must become a part of your lifestyle.

Let me list some slightly more focused, intentional lifestyle changes that can be very helpful if your goal is to lose weight.[8]

1. Get rid of some of the stress in your life before you focus on your weight. Clean up a few of the financial obligations that keep you worried, resolve relationship conflicts you are having, and practice better time-management strategies.

2. Make a list of what helps you to stay motivated and focused. Maybe it's a couple of hours of personal time each weekend or a relaxing walk on the beach. Or maybe there are Scripture verses or meaningful quotes that help to level out your emotions when stress sets in. Find a way to do these things during moments of temptation.

3. Pick some people who will support and encourage you in positive ways. Look for individuals who will not shame or embarrass you but will listen to your concerns and feelings and spend time creating healthy menus or sharing relaxing moments with you.

4. Set realistic goals. How do you know what is realistic? Generally it's best to aim for a loss of one to two pounds a week. Of course, to do that you need to consistently burn more calories (about one thousand extra each week), which you can do by getting regular exercise.

5. Learn to enjoy the real food you are eating. Eat tasty, interesting combinations of foods, and try new and different ways of preparing the food you eat.

6. Get active and stay active. This doesn't have to mean spending hours in a gym every week. Something as simple

as a brisk thirty-minute walk each day will provide steady aerobic exercise and will also be enjoyable.

7. Take a good look at your eating habits and daily routine. Try creating a strategy to gradually change your unhealthy habits and attitudes that may have led to failure in the past. Choose ways to maintain these new habits so you can succeed in losing weight for good.

LEARN TO LOVE THE BODY YOU HAVE

Even if you lose tons of weight, if you do not learn to love the person you are—inside and out—you will find it difficult to move forward in positive, motivating, and joyful ways. At my lowest point—overweight, filled with depression, overwhelmed with grief over the loss of my sister, and faced with the pain of not being able to give my newborn son the breast milk I knew would be so good for him—I no longer even liked myself. I liked nothing at all about who I was in those moments. I felt paralyzed, like I would never be able to move to a more positive place in my life. I would have been able to find ten things wrong with me for every one thing I could find right.

Unless you learn to love the person you are, just the way you are, you won't have the ability to make the necessary adjustments to achieve your dreams. You won't even be able to create that dream of a better you in your mind.

So how do we learn to love ourselves just as we are? One of the best things we can do is stop trying to emulate the images of the perfect body we see in magazines, on television, or in movies. Most of us—about 99 percent of us—will never be able to look like those models and celebrities we see in social media. The truth is, models and celebrities aren't as perfect as they seem. As *Experience Life* magazine noted, they often have been "professionally lit, professionally made up, professionally posed, and—by the time you see their photographs, professionally digitally retouched."[9]

> Unless you learn to love the person you are, just the way you are, you won't have the ability to make the necessary adjustments to achieve your dreams.

Recognize that it is not healthy to always be thinking, "If only I could look like her/him, then I could be happy and successful." Take your focus off trying to be someone else and focus on being the best you can be, just the way you are. Start thinking about the wonderful way the Creator made you. Hidden inside of you are all the tools and abilities you will ever need to be blown away by the big dreams you can achieve if you just say, "I can do it." I like to focus on a verse from Scripture that says, "Thank you for making me so wonderfully complex! It is amazing to think about. Your workmanship is marvelous—and how well I know it" (Ps. 139:14). Start realizing the potential you already have inside to dream big and to achieve those dreams.

> Beauty is not a physical state but a state of mind.

I want to suggest ten steps you can take to embrace a more positive body image. You can't automatically turn your negative thinking about yourself into a positive body image. But by faithfully following some of these simple steps recommended by the National Eating Disorders Association, you will learn to love the person you are, just the way you are.[10]

1. Appreciate all that your body can do. Every day your body carries you closer to your dreams. Celebrate all of the amazing things your body does for you—running, dancing, breathing, laughing, dreaming, etc.

2. Keep a top ten list of things you like about yourself—things that aren't related to how much you weigh or what you look like. Read your list often. Add to it as you become aware of more things to like about yourself.

3. Remind yourself that true beauty is not skin deep. When you feel good about yourself and who you are, you carry yourself with a sense of confidence, self-acceptance, and openness that makes you beautiful regardless of whether you physically look like a supermodel. Beauty is a state of mind, not a state of your body.

4. Look at yourself as a whole person. When you see yourself in a mirror or in your mind, choose not to focus on specific body parts. See yourself as you want others to see you—as a whole person.

5. Surround yourself with positive people. It is easier to feel good about yourself and your body when you are around supportive people who recognize the importance of liking yourself just as you naturally are.

6. Shut down those voices in your head that tell you your body is not "right" or that you are a "bad" person. You can overpower those negative thoughts with positive ones. The next time you start to tear yourself down, build yourself back up with a few quick affirmations that work for you.

AFFIRMATIONS FOR DEFEATING NEGATIVE THOUGHTS[11]

"I possess the qualities needed to be extremely successful."

"My ability to conquer my challenges is limitless; my potential to succeed is infinite."

"I am courageous and I stand up for myself."

"Today, I abandon my old habits and take up new, more positive ones."

"My fears of tomorrow are simply melting away."

7. Wear clothes that are comfortable and that make you feel good about your body. Work with your body, not against it.

8. Become a critical viewer of social and media messages. Pay attention to images, slogans, or attitudes that make you feel bad about yourself or your body. Protest these messages: write a letter to the advertiser or talk back to the image or message.

9. Do something nice for yourself—something that lets your body know you appreciate it. Take a bubble bath, make time for a nap, or find a peaceful place outside to relax.

10. Use the time and energy you might have spent worrying about food, calories, and your weight to do something to help others. Sometimes reaching out to other people can help you feel better about yourself and make a positive change in our world.

I have finally learned to love *me* just as I am. I'm fully content being who I am, doing what I do, dreaming of even bigger achievements, and spending quality time with my family, whom I love so much.

I'm an everyday natural person. I have an everyday natural body that is strong and capable and just right. I stay that way by eating an everyday natural diet of real food and by staying enjoyably active—whether that means working out hard on my exercise bike or gardening, raising chickens, turkeys, ducks, geese, rabbits, goats, sheep, cows, and who knows what next. I do it by spending countless hours playing with my kids, spending time with my husband, and going fun places with my family. I do it by being *me*—not someone else, just me. And being "just me" is perfectly all right with me.

> I'm fully content being who I am, doing what I do, dreaming of even bigger achievements, and spending quality time with my family, whom I love so much.

Start making the food choices that will lead you to conquer once and for all that battle with the bulge. And while you are losing weight and bringing your body to a healthier state, concentrate also on learning to have a better body image that allows you to love the person you are, just the way you are. Then you too will be able to dream big and achieve those dreams.

Chapter 7

EMBRACING
NATURAL HYGIENE

I REMEMBER WHEN MY sister and I reached our teen years and began earning money by babysitting and doing odd jobs. Suddenly we had a little money of our own, and we could be in charge of how we spent it. Sure, a small portion of it went for Cokes and chips, but like true girls, we mostly wanted to buy the latest beauty lotions, shampoos, and colognes. Before long the two of us had just about every beauty or body product that was trending.

We really didn't know, or care, what was in those products. We just bought them because they either smelled good, looked good on us, or promised some lasting effect that we thought we desperately needed.

At some point I started hearing that some of these products were not all that safe. They were filled with all kinds of toxic chemicals and unsafe additives. Maybe it was when I heard that my glamorous, shiny eye makeup was filled with fish gills, or when, being a real animal lover, I heard how the big beauty product companies used animals to test their products, which caused cancers in the animals, that I started thinking about whether these products were actually safe for me. After some research I decided it was time to purge my drawers and dresser tops of these dangerous products and start using more natural alternatives.

I lost my confidence in the Food and Drug Administration (FDA) to keep me safe when I read that only 11 percent of the thousands of ingredients the FDA says are safe had actually been assessed for safety.[1] I recommend that you do some independent research of your own if you are still using over-the-counter bath and beauty products. A good place to start is the Holistic Health Magazine & Resource Directory.[2]

ELIMINATE THE DANGEROUS CHEMICALS

In your journey to a more natural lifestyle, hygiene will be an important area to confront. So many of the products we use are connected to us emotionally—they fulfill our desires to look good, smell good, and be attractive, especially to the opposite sex. We try to emulate what movie and TV beauty icons use to look *soooo* glamorous.

But those body-care products often are filled with toxic chemicals that have absolutely no benefit to anyone. In fact, many of them can have detrimental effects on us. It is sad but true that most of the bath and beauty products you can buy in stores are filled with unhealthy chemicals and additives. Consider the following.

1. *Body lotions*—Many over-the-counter body lotions contain "fragrance," which could be one of more than two hundred different chemicals that do not have to be disclosed by the companies making them. These "fragrances" are junk food for your skin and can cause problems such as rash, dizziness, headaches, vomiting, hyperpigmentation, skin irritations, and even cancer.[3]

2. *Mouthwash*—Many people use mouthwash to keep their teeth, gums, and tongues feeling fresh and clean. But we are often just swishing around a mouthful of harsh, dangerous chemicals. Mouthwash contains alcohol, which dries and changes the pH of the mouth and throat, and has been linked with an increased risk of mouth and throat cancers. It also contains fluoride, sorbitol, and saccharin, which has caused bladder cancer in test animals. Mouthwash also carries the same dangerous fragrances as body lotions.[4]

3. *Antiperspirant deodorants*—It's pretty obvious that we all need a good deodorant! The more we sweat, the more we stink. But many antiperspirants actually prevent perspiration from occurring by using aluminum as the active ingredient. Aluminum, a known neurotoxin, is harmful to your body. A number of health issues are associated with it, including breast cancer, kidney problems, bone conditions, and Alzheimer's disease.[5]

The best way to move to safer, more natural body and beauty products is to learn to read the ingredient lists carefully. There are many chemicals and additives to avoid. For example, many hygiene care products include both synthetic and organic versions of these five ingredients: emollients, humectants, emulsifiers, surfactants, and preservatives.[6] Though known to be dangerous, many of these chemicals continue to be used regularly in over-the-counter products. Here is a list of twenty toxins to avoid:[7]

- Coal tar, a known carcinogen, has been banned in Europe but is still used in North America. You can find it in dry skin treatments and shampoos designed to resist lice and dandruff. It is typically listed as a color with a number, such as FD&C Red No. 6.

- DEA/TEA/MEA may be carcinogens and are used in shampoos, body washes, and soaps as emulsifiers.

- Ethoxylated surfactants and 1,4-dioxane are never listed; 1,4-dioxane is a by-product created when carcinogenic ethylene oxide is added to other chemicals. The Environmental Working Group (EWG) has found 1,4-dioxane in 57 percent of baby washes in the United States. As a general rule, stay away from ingredients that contain the letters *eth*.

- Formaldehyde is a suspected carcinogen and irritant and can be found in nail products and in some makeup. It is banned in Europe.

- Fragrance/parfum is a catchall phrase for hidden chemicals. Fragrance is also known to cause headaches, asthma, allergies, and dizziness.

- Hydroquinone is used for lightening skin. It is banned in England and is rated toxic on the EWG's Skin Deep database. It has been linked to cancer.

- Lead, a known carcinogen, is found in some lipstick and hair dye. It is considered a contaminant and not an ingredient, so it is never listed on labels.

- Mercury is a known allergen that negatively impacts brain development. It is found in makeup and even in some eye drops.

- Mineral oil is a by-product of petroleum and is used in baby oil, moisturizers, and a variety of styling gels. The film it leaves can hamper the skin's ability to release toxins.

- Oxybenzone, the active ingredient in chemical-based sunscreens, collects in fatty tissues. It is linked to hormone disruption, allergies, low birth weight, and cellular damage.

- Parabens, which are used as preservatives, are included in many products. They may contribute to cancer, reproductive toxicity, and endocrine disruption.

- Paraphenylenediamine (PPD), though used in hair products and dyes, is very toxic to the skin and immune system.

- Phthalates are man-made chemicals that are mainly used as plasticizers (meaning they are added to plastics to increase their flexibility and durability). Though banned in children's toys in Europe and California, they can be found in many perfumes, lotions, and deodorants. They are linked to endocrine disruption, cancer, and damage to liver, kidney, and lung function.

- Placental extract is a substance used in some skin and hair products. It is linked to disruption of the endocrine system.

- Polyethylene glycol (PEG) is used in many products to enhance penetration. It is often contaminated with 1,4-dioxane and ethylene oxide, which were listed earlier as carcinogens.

- Silicone-derived emollients are added to make a product feel soft. These are not biodegradable and are linked both to skin irritation and the growth of tumors.

- Sodium lauryl (ether) sulfate (SLS, SLES) was formerly used as an industrial degreaser and is now used to make soap foamy. The body absorbs this chemical, and it is known to irritate the skin.

- Talc, which is similar to asbestos, can be found in baby powder, deodorant, blush, and even eye shadow. Sadly it has been linked to ovarian cancer and respiratory issues.

+ Toluene, which disrupts the endocrine and immune systems, also affects fetal development. It is used in nail and hair products.

+ Triclosan is found in antibacterial products, deodorants, and hand sanitizers. It has been linked to cancer and endocrine disruption.[8]

CHOOSE A MORE NATURAL WAY

If you are anxious to rid your body of some of the dangerous chemicals and additives used in conventional hygiene products, there are three primary healthy, natural ways to do this: buying organic, making your own natural hygiene products, and using essential oils. In this section I want to take a look at each of these options and, I hope, help you find ways to use healthier hygiene products.

Buy organic, natural hygiene products

Many people are working hard today to find safer, healthier products to use for their natural hygiene needs. If that describes you, one place to start is getting to know the organic skin care and beauty products available in many of the stores where you already shop and in health-conscious retailers. By learning to recognize unhealthy and dangerous product chemicals and tell the difference between synthetic and natural ingredients, you will be prepared to make wise choices about organic skin- and body-care products. With some simple online research, you can become very familiar with the natural, organic ingredients you want to see listed on the products you use.

There are so many benefits to making the transition to natural, organic hygiene products. Some of the best benefits are noted in the following list developed by blogger Stephanie Petersen:[9]

+ Natural products are earth-friendly. The ingredients in natural health and beauty products release far fewer chemicals into the air and water.

+ Natural products save your nose from artificial fragrances that can cause some people to experience headaches. Natural health and beauty products scented with quality essential oils can even provide aromatherapy.

- Natural products are gentler and have no strange side effects, unlike their chemical-laden counterparts. Natural health and beauty products use natural preservatives, such as grapefruit seed extract, that won't affect your body or cause irritation.

As you consider which skin- and body-care products to buy, it is important to remember this one thing: what you put on your body is important to your health. Using toxic ingredients could be the final barrier to great health. Eliminating these toxins could lead to the better outcome you've been seeking.

Remember that some harmful ingredients are not listed in conventionally made products. To be sure you are safe, stick with organic bath and body products.

Make your own natural hygiene products

I began my journey to natural health out of desperate need. I was broken down—body, soul, and spirit. With each step I've taken, my joy, peace, and positive thinking and acting has grown by leaps and bounds.

I have enjoyed finding that I could even make some of the organic, natural hygiene products that would maximize my family's health. In later chapters I will talk about natural ways to care for your face, hair, and body. In this section I concentrate on oral health products that are easy to make at home to support better health.

> As you consider which skin- and body-care products to buy, it is important to remember this one thing: what you put on your body is important to your health.

I began looking for natural solutions a couple of years ago. I went to the dentist for what I thought was going to be a routine cleaning and was horrified to walk out with a hefty quote for dental work that needed to be done on *six* cavities the dentist found in my teeth.

At first I was embarrassed. Shocked. I eat a very clean, whole foods diet. How could I have cavities? I don't even eat white sugar. I brush and floss every day! How could this be true?

I told my dentist that I don't eat sugar or complex carbs and asked him if there was a way I could heal my cavities without having thousands of dollars of dental work done. I told him I had heard of "remineralizing" and curing tooth decay with diet and asked him what he thought. Of course, like many conventional dentists, he had never heard of it. So I stopped asking questions, grabbed my quote, scheduled an appointment to have all six cavities filled, and went home discouraged.

When I got home I started reading and researching natural ways to heal your teeth. I read the book *Cure Tooth Decay: Remineralize Cavities and Repair Your Teeth Naturally With Good Food*, and my mind was blown.[10] I thought, "I can heal my cavities without having thousands of dollars of dental work done? I can heal my cavities with proper diet? I can remineralize my teeth? I'm in!"

To fully understand how to heal my cavities, I had to know what was the root cause of my tooth decay. Here is what I found: in a 1915 landmark study of groups from around the world, Dr. Weston A. Price discovered that the root cause of tooth decay is the lack of healthy nutrients in the modern diet.[11] So after doing more extensive research into the possibility of healing my own tooth decay, I began making the following healthy choices:

+ I take 1 teaspoon of extra-virgin fermented cod liver oil* daily.

+ I take 1 teaspoon of high-vitamin butter oil* daily.

+ I take 1 teaspoon of skate liver oil* (a type of fish oil) daily.

+ I drink three to four cups of raw milk (goat's or cow's) each day.

+ I drink one cup of homemade bone stock each day and use grass-fed beef gelatin to cook with and add to beverages.

+ I eat liver once a week. If this grosses you out, you can take desiccated liver tablets.

+ I use liberal amounts of grass-fed butter and ghee in my foods and recipes. However, this is *not* to be considered a substitute for high-vitamin butter oil, which is extracted from butter without the use of heat.

+ I oil pull with coconut oil. Not sure what oil pulling is? I swish about a tablespoon of coconut oil in my mouth on an empty stomach for around twenty minutes. This can help draw toxins out of your body and improve your overall health, not just your oral health. If you want to know more about oil pulling, I recommend you read *Oil Pulling Therapy* by Bruce Fife.[12]

+ I avoid any toothpaste with glycerin, as it counteracts remineralization. I make my own toothpaste using bentonite clay, or I buy an organic, natural brand. (See my recipe in this chapter.)

I normally don't eat many grains, plant seeds, or other foods high in phytic acid (which may neutralize the absorption of iron, zinc, and calcium, and may promote mineral deficiencies). If I do eat grains, I make sure they are traditionally prepared (by soaking, sprouting, or souring). I also make sure my nut butters come from a trustworthy source and are soaked before being pureed. If you are not willing to give up your grains, look into taking a vitamin C supplement to help neutralize the phytic acid.

DIY Remineralizing Toothpaste

⅓ cup bentonite clay (This comes from pure sources of undisturbed deposits in the ground and draws toxins out of the body.)
¼ cup boiling water
1 Tbsp. coconut oil (Coconut oil is amazing for oral health. It is highly effective with getting rid of viruses and bacteria in the mouth.)
¼ tsp. real salt (Real salt is unrefined and full of natural minerals.)
½ tsp. real stevia (the dry herb that is green and unprocessed)
15 drops of Protective Blend essential oil
10 drops of peppermint essential oil

Put your bentonite clay in a bowl. Heat the water on the stove and then stir in the coconut oil till it is melted. With a hand mixer, mix on medium speed the bentonite clay and the water/oil mixture till blended through. Add the salt, stevia, and essential oils and continue to blend until it is completely blended. Keep in a covered jar!

The mixture will harden a little bit as it sits because of the coconut oil. This makes it easier to add a bit to your toothbrush when you brush.

Use essential oils for natural hygiene

Essential oils are volatile aromatic compounds extracted from plants, fruit, seeds, roots, and bark, and they have powerful health benefits. They can be used for a wide array of purposes for your health, home, and homemade recipes. However, not all essential oils are the same. In fact, many are synthetic and will do nothing for your health. When you buy essential oils, you must be sure they are 100 percent pure therapeutic grade. Be vigilant to do your research.

Using essential oils to support your health is called aromatherapy, and natural-minded, holistic people have been doing this for thousands of years. When essential oils enter the bloodstream, they have an effect on the whole body. They can enter the bloodstream through various application methods (diffusing, topical use, or internal use), and then circulate through the bloodstream and interact with tissues and cells throughout the body.

MY HOMEMADE HERBAL MOUTHWASH

My Instagram followers know that I wore Invisalign braces a few years ago to straighten my teeth. Having the braces on my teeth twenty-two hours a day made my mouth stale and dry. I am a minimalist, and before braces I would just brush my teeth then drop a little bit of peppermint essential oil on my tongue and swish it around. However, with the braces, I needed something that would swish really well and freshen my breath, which is why I created this herbal mouthwash. I'm now sort of addicted to it, and I know you will be too!

DIY HERBAL MOUTHWASH

2 cups filtered water

2 Tbsp. dried peppermint leaves

10 drops of therapeutic-grade peppermint essential oil*

5–10 drops of therapeutic-grade cinnamon essential oil* (you decide how much)

½ tsp. vitamin C powder (to act as a preservative)

Put the water in a small pot and bring it to a simmer. Add the peppermint leaves, reduce the heat, cover, and simmer for fifteen minutes. Use a cheesecloth to strain the herbs, and cool. Add the essential oils and vitamin C powder. Store in a glass jar and shake before each use. You will be amazed at the fresh, clean, healthy way your mouth feels from your continual use of this mouthwash.

America is a little late to the essential oils game and is just now becoming aware of the many benefits essential oils can bring to our bodies. Following are the top five essential oils and their benefits in natural hygiene.

Lavender

People have loved using lavender for thousands of years because of its unmistakable aroma and beneficial properties. Its primary benefits include soothing occasional skin irritations, helping to reduce anxious feelings because of its high amount of linalool, promoting a peaceful night's sleep, and easing feelings of tension.

Lavender is commonly used in many DIY natural body-care products, but there are many ways to use lavender essential oil. I would suggest these three uses: (1) add a few drops of lavender oil to your pillow or feet at bedtime; (2) keep a bottle of lavender oil on hand to soothe occasional skin irritations; (3) add lavender oil to a roll-on bottle and top with fractionated coconut oil (a form of the oil that remains liquid at room temperature and doesn't clog pores)[13] and apply to wrists, neck, and feet to help reduce feelings of stress.

One of my favorite uses for lavender oil is to make a luxurious body butter. I have to admit, I have an obsession with making body butter. There's something about putting together the simplest of ingredients and then whipping them up into a natural, nourishing lotion. My Lavender Body Butter does just that, and it's simple to make. You can find the recipe in chapter 10.

Frankincense

Cherished as one of the most precious essential oils, frankincense has remarkable health benefits. It is particularly soothing and rejuvenating for the skin. Some of its other primary benefits include promoting healthy cellular function and feelings of relaxation, helping to balance the mood, and reducing the appearance of skin imperfections.

Try using it in these ways: apply to the bottoms of your feet or diffuse to promote feelings of relaxation and help to balance mood, or add one to two drops to skin to reduce the appearance of skin imperfections.

Melaleuca

More commonly known as tea tree oil, melaleuca essential oil has more than ninety different compounds and limitless applications. Some of its primary benefits include helping to maintain healthy immune function, protecting against environmental and seasonal threats, and cleansing and rejuvenating the skin.

Here are some of the ways you can use this beneficial essential oil. For occasional skin irritations, apply one to two drops of melaleuca on the affected area. Apply a few drops to a spray bottle and mix with water, and spray on surfaces to protect against environmental threats. You can also combine one to two drops with your facial cleanser or apply to skin after shaving for extra benefit.

Peppermint

The peppermint plant is a hybrid of the watermint and spearmint plants and is an oil I could not live without. It is extremely beneficial as it promotes healthy respiratory function, clear breathing, and digestive health, and it is a natural bug repellant.

Some of the many ways to use peppermint oil include using a drop of peppermint in water for a healthy, refreshing mouthwash; rubbing it on top of your stomach to help alleviate occasional stomach upset; or placing one drop in the palms of your hands and inhaling it for a midday pick-me-up.

Lemon

Lemon is the top-selling essential oil and has multiple benefits and uses. Its powerful cleansing properties help to purify the air and surfaces, and it can be used as a nontoxic cleaner throughout the home. It is also a natural cleanser for the body, aids in digestion, and helps to promote a positive mood.

Try adding lemon oil to a spray bottle and spraying it on surfaces, tables, sinks, and countertops. Or diffuse it in your home to create an uplifting environment—or *natural hygiene for the home!*

The most important thing to know about essential oils is that they are not all created equal. Where a plant is grown has a major impact on its constitution, which then determines the potency of the plant. Another important factor is when the plant is harvested and what part of the plant is selected. Both play a major role in determining the quality of an essential oil. This is why I carefully choose the essential oils I use from a reputable, quality company.[14] This organization is a step above any other essential oil brand I have ever used. They have very strict testing standards and harvest their oils all over the world from each plant's prime environment.[15]

NOW IT'S YOUR TURN TO GET MOVING

Once you begin making the transition to organic, natural hygiene products, you will find that you are becoming healthier by freeing your body of the dangerous, toxic chemicals and additives found in the majority of traditional products available today. However, you may make the same mistake I did by deciding to completely revamp your hygiene routine by purchasing all the latest natural products on the market. Start small. Eliminate the most dangerous over-the-counter traditional products and find one or two organic natural products that will cover several needs.

It won't take long for you to discover that this can be a real budget-breaking move on your part. You may be spending nearly as much on these products as you do on your weekly groceries—and that's a mistake none of us can afford.

I recommend that you keep these super cost-efficient products on hand: coconut oil, raw apple cider vinegar, raw honey, sea salt, and sugar. These inexpensive products can be used in many home-made hygiene products. If you lack the confidence to develop your own recipes, there are hundreds of wonderful homemade natural hygiene product recipes online.

As you journey to live a more natural lifestyle, the key is to start somewhere and keep moving forward. You will find making your own hygiene products to be so much fun, and so fulfilling, that you will never look back.

Chapter 8

RADIANT SKIN

$\mathcal{A}$RE YOU AWARE that your skin is your body's largest organ? Experts have determined that it takes more than 18.5 square feet of skin to cover our flesh and bones, with skin making up 16 percent of our body weight.[1] Our skin is vitally important in ensuring good health. So it stands to reason that one of the most important ways we can be successful on our journey to health is to understand how to adequately care for our skin.

Here are just a few of the things we need to know about our skin and its care:[2]

+ Your skin plays a key role in regulating body temperature. It is your body's thermostat. In higher temperatures sweat glands activate to cool your body down. In cooler temperatures your pores become smaller in order to retain heat.

+ Your skin regenerates itself. Dead skin cells are shed daily, and a new layer of skin is created every twenty-eight days. That is one of the reasons why it is so important to support the removal of dead skin cells with an exfoliator.

+ Millions of bacteria known as microbiota live on the skin. These harmless bacteria help your immune cells fight microbes, which cause disease.

+ Your skin can reveal many things about your health. Rashes, hives, or itching may be signals of an allergic response, a bacterial or viral infection, or even an autoimmune disease. Changes in a mole should be taken seriously, as they may be an indication of skin cancer.

Taking good care of your skin involves both what you put on your body (topical applications) and what you put in it (ideally, beneficial natural foods). In this chapter I want to give you some information that will help you begin to care for your skin more naturally. I will include some healthy, natural protocols for your skin, scalp, and hair to help you keep your skin healthy and glowing for years to come.

THE BASICS OF NATURAL SKIN CARE

On our journey to better natural health, we have been learning to transition from products laden with dangerous chemicals and additives to natural, organic products. But there are both good and bad natural products. Top skin care experts have identified which natural ingredients and protocols have proven to be the most effective in helping people achieve the healthiest, most radiant skin possible. These natural ingredients and protocols include the following.

Beta-carotene

Red, orange, and yellow fruits and vegetables are loaded with beta-carotene. Your body converts beta-carotene into vitamin A, which is essential for protecting against sun damage, healing wounds, and encouraging cell turnover.[3] Topical natural products with beta-carotene also have antioxidant benefits for your skin.

I want to give you two recipes that will help you add beta-carotene to your skin care routine. One recipe is a smoothie that will allow you to ingest beta-carotene, and the other is a beta-carotene–rich exfoliant you can apply topically to get rid of dead skin cells.

Spirulina Smoothie

Spirulina is one of the top superfoods. This blue-green vegetable algae is a freshwater plant that has been used as a source of nutrition for centuries. It has the highest levels of protein and beta-carotene of all the green superfoods. It is also the vegetable with the highest known level of B_{12}. Spirulina is easy to digest, protects the immune system, supports mineral absorption, and helps regulate cholesterol.[4] I like to add it to my post-workout smoothie. You can add it to any smoothie any way you like, but this is my favorite recipe.

10–12 oz. of coconut water
1 Tbsp. chia seeds

1–2 Tbsp. spirulina (start small and increase over time)
1 frozen banana
1–2 cups frozen berries
1–2 scoops of your favorite protein powder (optional)

Throw everything in the blender and blend till smooth! I don't need to add a sweetener because the banana and berries are usually enough for me. If you find you need a little sweetening, add some stevia or raw honey. Oh, and I have to make a little extra for my two kiddos—they have no idea how healthy this is! Your skin—and your kids—will love you for giving them that extra boost of beta-carotene.

Pumpkin Sugar Scrub Bars

Sugar scrubs are fantastic for sloughing off dead skin cells. As a bonus, they lather up great and leave you feeling so refreshed after you use them.

I like to make mine in bars, which I form by using silicone muffin pans. These Pumpkin Sugar Scrub Bars will provide the beta-carotene your skin needs and are so refreshing to use.

1 cup white sugar
1 cup brown sugar
10 drops each of ginger, cinnamon, and eucalyptus essential oils*
1 cup pumpkin puree
2 tsp. vanilla
2 Tbsp. honey

Mix the sugars in a bowl. Add remaining ingredients and mix well. Scoop the mixture evenly into eight silicone muffin molds. Freeze for 20–30 minutes, and you are done! I keep mine in the fridge during the summer months, when my house is warmer. When you are ready to shower, grab a bar and lather up! Your skin is going to love you.

Green tea extract

Green tea has high levels of antioxidant chemicals that help prevent or even reverse UV damage to the skin. It is often used in skin care for its excellent natural anti-inflammatory and skin-soothing properties.[5] Green tea may also slow the skin-aging process and prevent premature dry skin from causing your skin to lose its radiance.[6] There are several ways you can incorporate green tea into your skin-care routine. Try some of the following:

+ Switch to drinking green tea instead of black tea. After each cup of green tea you make, cut the tea bag open and empty it into a small cup. Add a little honey to make it into a paste, and apply the paste to your freshly cleaned face. Leave the mask on for ten minutes then rinse it off.

+ Let a cup of freshly brewed green tea cool for a few minutes. When it is cooler, pour some tea into your hand and splash it over your face. Repeat until there is no more tea. Rinse your face with cool water.

+ Use matcha green tea powder to make a green tea facial mask. Matcha is a superfood and can boost detoxification and immunity, help to reduce inflammation, and even skin tone. Mix a teaspoon of matcha green tea powder with about a teaspoon of raw honey and stir to form a paste. Spread over your face and leave on ten or fifteen minutes before removing with a warm, wet washcloth.[7]

Oil cleansing

Over time I've traded in my expensive over-the-counter facial products for simple and natural ingredients. Not only are the ingredients I use 100 percent natural, but they are also safer and more effective than anything I could purchase from the store. But it's not just the ingredients that are making a difference.

For a while now I have been doing the oil cleansing method for my facial skin care, and I must say, I will *never* go back to buying any other form of facial cleansing product. I know it may seem absurd to throw oil on an already oily face to clean it, but oil cleanses oil. Oil moisturizes. Oil softens. Oil is natural, made by the earth. Oil has *one* ingredient—oil.

There are several kinds of oil you can use as a facial cleanser. I use a mixture of jojoba and castor oil. Castor oil is an amazing cleansing agent. I put the oil mixture in an old glass bottle and shake it up before I use it.

When it's time to cleanse my face, I splash some water on my face and put a quarter-size amount of the oil mixture on my hand. Then I rub the oil all over my face and into my pores in a circular motion. Next, I get a washcloth and put it under hot water. I lay the washcloth over my face and let the steam open my pores. (You're supposed to keep it on for about a minute or so, but I am usually in such a hurry to get myself ready that it only stays on my face for a couple of seconds.) Then I take the washcloth and rub the oil into my skin.

> I've been using the oil cleansing method on my face for years. I love it and rarely use even natural, organic cleansers or moisturizers.

I use circular motions again and rub the oil off. I do this until all the oil is absorbed into my pores as much as possible and my face is no longer oily. I pat dry with a towel, and I'm done! My face is soft and never needs anything more! I do this every night, and I just splash water on my face in the mornings. I have been using the oil cleansing method on my face for years. I love it and rarely use even natural, organic cleansers or moisturizers.

Here is a list of some of the most effective carrier oils to use to cleanse your face developed by a blogger known as Crunchy Betty:[8]

- Argan oil (good for all skin types, especially aging skin, but it's pricey)
- Avocado oil (good for dry and aging skin)
- Grapeseed oil (good for all skin types, particularly especially oily skin)
- Jojoba oil (good for all skin types but very desirable for acne-prone skin)
- Sunflower seed oil (good for all skin types)
- Sweet almond oil (good for all skin types, particularly especially oily skin)
- Tamanu oil (good for all skin types but also very pricey)

To cleanse your face, mix an equal part of one of these carrier oils with castor oil. (If your skin is dry, use one-third castor oil and two-thirds carrier oil; if your skin is oily, do the opposite: use one-third carrier oil and two-thirds castor oil.)[9] Rinse your face lightly with warm water. Pour the oil in the palm of your hand and gently apply to your face using circular motions for about two minutes. You can let the oils just sit on your face for another minute. Or if you're in a hurry, as I usually am, you can just soak a washcloth in hot water and hold it to your face for ten to fifteen seconds. Then slowly wipe the oil off your skin.

> I haven't used traditional shampoo, conditioner, or hair products on my hair in a long time. My hair has never felt so amazing. It's soft and shiny, and it is healthy.

Antiaging essential oils

Lately, as I'm getting a tad bit older, I have been using specific antiaging essential oils to help promote healthy skin. I created a DIY Facial Serum that uses my favorite essential oils that are known for their antiaging benefits. I use:

+ *Lavender*—Lavender is great for all skin types but very powerful for mature skin. It is widely known for its calming and relaxing properties but is also great for soothing mild skin irritations.

+ *Frankincense*—Frankincense is one of the most valued essential oils. It is used in many beauty products to slow the signs of aging and to promote youthful, radiant skin.

+ *Geranium*—Geranium essential oil has been used since the days of ancient Egypt to beautify skin. It helps to give you clear, healthy skin and is an ideal ingredient for skin care products.

+ *Myrrh*—Myrrh was so prized in ancient times that at times it was valued at its weight in gold. It is also soothing to the skin, promoting a smooth, youthful-looking complexion.

DIY Facial Serum

50 ml glass dropper bottle (old stevia dropper
bottles are great for things like this)
4 Tbsp. of almond or jojoba oil (or one of
the other beneficial cleansing oils listed
previously)
7 drops each of lavender, frankincense,
geranium, and myrrh essential oils
The contents of 2 capsules of vitamin E

Add all the ingredients to your dropper bottle
and shake well. Apply this serum to your face
each night before you go to bed.

NATURAL PROTOCOLS FOR YOUR SCALP AND HAIR

There are many natural methods you can use to clean your hair instead of using the heavily perfumed and chemical-laden shampoos and conditioners sold in stores. I want to recommend a couple of options for you, and I would challenge you to do your own research and experiment with some of the many natural methods for caring for your scalp and hair.

Traditional vs. organic shampoo

Liquid shampoo was invented in Germany in 1927.[10] Before that, people used bars of shampoo soap. Liquid shampoos generated lots of suds, but creating suds meant using synthetic surfactants (detergents that create foam). These synthetic additives include *diethanolamine* (DEA), which can result in eye and skin irritation;[11] *formaldehyde*, also an irritant and known carcinogen;[12] and *sulfates*. Sulfates create lather, but they may damage the hair and cause scalp irritation.[13] Many shampoos also contain *isopropyl alcohol* or other petroleum derivatives, which help the hair to *look* clean but actually strip it of important proteins and take away natural moisture.[14] Additional additives such as fragrances, colorings, and preservatives are all toxic.[15]

I haven't used traditional shampoo, conditioner, or hair products on my hair in a long time. My hair has never felt so amazing. It's soft and shiny, and it is healthy.

Organic shampoos use ingredients such as tea tree products, which have great benefits for the skin and scalp; beta-glucan, which soothes the scalp; and aloe vera, coconut oil, and shea butter, which are all natural moisturizers.

Traditional shampoos contain a lot of artificial ingredients that can have negative effects on the hair and scalp. Skin irritations often occur, and there are negative effects when the chemicals are absorbed into your body. These artificial ingredients need to be used in order to allow the shampoo to foam and create suds. Without foam and suds, many people do not believe the shampoo is working.

Conventional shampoos also strip hair of the natural oils so necessary for healthy hair. Instead they often deposit oils that make the hair look greasy. Organic shampoos use healthy, natural oils that leave hair soft and silky. Although organic shampoo is usually a little pricier, it sure makes all the difference in healthy hair and scalp conditions.[16]

How to choose natural, organic skin and hair products

As with most things in life, the idea that "any old natural shampoo will do" is just not true. When you are choosing the products that will be used on your skin and scalp, you need to know how to choose the safest nontoxic products available. Here are a few simple steps you can take:[17]

+ *Stick with just the basics*—A safe, natural product needs only basic ingredients.

+ *Be sure you know what you are really getting*—Examine product labels carefully. The words *natural* and *all-natural* are not regulated labeling terms.

+ *Say no to fragrance*—Dozens of toxic chemicals may be mixed in a single product's fragrance mixture. Use unscented products.

+ *Choose packaging that can be recycled*—The ideal option is glass because it is recyclable and won't leach toxins into the product.

+ *Choose products made with organic ingredients*—This includes those grown without synthetic fertilizers or pesticides, and botanicals grown using biodynamic farming methods. Look for the Demeter USA stamp of approval on the label. Demeter International is the only certifier of biodynamic farms and products in the world.[18]

+ *Sidestep the petrochemicals*—These are obtained from natural gas and are identified on labels as *petrolatum, mineral oil,* and *paraffin.*

+ *Ignore exotic trends*—Every so often a trend will emerge promising to be the answer to all your skin-related problems, but often these trends cause serious damage to your skin, the environment, or both.

Homemade, natural shampoos

Many people today are opting to make their own natural, homemade shampoo. It is safer, and can be surprisingly budget-friendly and provide much better results than store-bought shampoos. You can find many recipes online for homemade shampoos.[19]

Natural rinses and conditioners

There are dozens and dozens of good DIY recipes for homemade conditioners available online. I have found that there is nothing quite as wonderful to rinse my hair with as a 50–50 mixture of apple cider vinegar and water. If you want to mask the smell of the vinegar, as I do, you can add a few drops of your favorite essential oil. I particularly like the scent of wild orange essential oil.

Making your own hair conditioner is a great way to target your hair's exact needs without the use of any unhealthy chemicals or additives. Many of us deal with frizzy, dry, or damaged hair from overtreating, overdrying, over-curling, or overprocessing our hair. Damaged hair can lead to split ends that limit hair growth and can cause your hair to lose its natural sheen and thickness.

There are simple, homemade conditioners you can make to remedy your damaged hair. You can make a simple healing conditioner using natural ingredients such as avocados, bananas, eggs, honey, and extra-virgin olive oil.

Healing Conditioner[20]

1 avocado
½ banana
1–2 Tbsp. olive oil

1 egg

Mash one avocado into a paste. Add the banana and olive oil to the paste. Using a blender, mix one egg into the avocado mixture until it is nice and soft. Apply to dry hair, starting with the top section of your hair (not your scalp) and working your way down to your hair tips. Concentrate on the tips, because that is where hair tends to suffer the most damage. Leave the conditioning paste on for about ten minutes and then rinse with water.

Natural hair dye

Henna* is the safest way to color your hair. It has been used for thousands of years to keep hair healthy and to color white or gray hair. Henna is a plant that grows in hot, dry climates. Its leaves are harvested, dehydrated, and then made into powder. When henna is mixed with an acid medium, it will stain your nails, skin, or hair into a reddish-brown color. This makes it a safe, nontoxic way to dye your hair. There is only *one* color of henna; however, there are different ranges of that color depending on the climate and soil of the particular henna plant.[21]

There are many amazing benefits to using henna. It is a natural, nontoxic coloring agent, a cure for head lice, and a cure for dandruff. It also leaves your hair silky, thick, and healthy, and provides therapeutic relief for headaches.[22]

> With just a little work on your part, you can maintain firm, youthful, radiant skin throughout your entire life.

I have been using henna to cover my gray for several years. Thanks to the genes from my mother, I began finding gray hair when I was just fifteen! Henna leaves my hair silky and smooth, and gives a red highlight to the gray hairs, but does not completely color all my hair.

Because it is important to use the right kind of henna and to be sure to apply it correctly, I refer you to my instructional blogs, which you can find at ThePaleoMama.com.[23]

With just a little work on your part, you can maintain strong, healthy hair and firm, youthful, radiant skin throughout your entire life.

One of the greatest benefits to our hair and skin is water. To ensure that your skin stays healthy, drink loads of water, taking small sips throughout your day. Water helps to plump up all your cells and keeps your skin looking firmer, more youthful, and radiant. Also, remember to eat foods that contribute to healthy skin and keep your stress at a minimum. The lower your stress level, the calmer you will be, and that will lead to a calm complexion that stays blemish-free.

Chapter 9

FINDING THE PATH TO NATURAL HEALTH

*M*ANY PEOPLE TODAY are dangerously unhealthy. Roughly two-thirds of American adults are overweight and more than a quarter are obese. Type 2 diabetes has affected as many as one in four Americans. As the number of Americans considered diabetic or prediabetic has skyrocketed, life expectancy has decreased. Conditions once considered rare—such as heart disease, stroke, cancer, and Alzheimer's disease—have become common and are even reaching near-epidemic levels.[1]

Even more worrying is the fact that Americans spend twice as much on health care as any other nation but rank last in the quality of care they receive. So the bottom line is that we spend more money to stay healthy, but our health is actually getting poorer.[2]

If we keep doing what we've been doing, we will keep seeing these horrible results—and worsening health. It is time for you to take responsibility for your own health. In this chapter I want to give you some simple tips and solutions that can help you and your family avoid illness and experience consistently good health.

Many of the things I recommend are homemade remedies I have developed for use in my own family. We have seen that using these natural, healthy solutions has enabled our family to avoid many of the illnesses that seem to spread rapidly at certain times of the year. Overall our health status has been positive, and we have been free of illness and disease consistently over several years.

TACKLING SEASONAL COLDS AND FLUS

Let's begin by taking a look at natural, homemade solutions for the annual seasonal respiratory distress and its associated problems. These are all great options for boosting immunity.

Soothing elixir

The moment I feel myself getting the sniffles, I grab a few lemons, some ginger, green tea, cinnamon, and local raw honey, and I make a soothing elixir to boost my immune system. It's so deeply nourishing and easy to make. You can make it in the slow cooker, let it simmer all day,

> It is time for you to take your health into your own hands.

and ladle a hot glass when you want it. Or you can make it on the stovetop. Either way works great, and there are many "add-ins" you can include to make it even more nutritious.

Soothing Cold Season Elixir

2 lemons, sliced in circles
8 tea bags
3 cinnamon sticks
2-inch-piece ginger, sliced thin
¼–½ cup raw apple cider vinegar
6 cups water
Raw honey to taste
Turmeric, coconut oil, or gelatin (optional)

Pour the water in a pot and bring to a boil. Add the lemons, ginger, tea bags, and cinnamon sticks. Cover and let steep for twenty to thirty minutes. Pour the apple cider vinegar into a pitcher or a large half-gallon Mason jar. Dump the tea into the Mason jar. You can leave in the lemons and ginger, but remove the tea bags. When the elixir is ready to drink, warm it up and add raw honey to taste.

Elderberry syrup

The elderberry plant is among the most sustainable crops and is being cultivated by many organic farmers. Elderberry fruit is packed with vitamins, minerals, and antioxidants. One of the best-known benefits of the black elderberry is its power to boost the immune system because of its strong antiviral properties. The medicinal parts of the elderberry bush include the roots, bark, young shoots, leaves, flowers, and berries. Yup—the entire plant![3]

Elderberry flowers are effective at reducing phlegm and encourage sweating. They are also good for strengthening the upper respiratory tract.[4] The flowers help to soften the skin and are often added to lotions and creams.[5]

Surprisingly most of the elderberry products marketed in the United States are actually grown in Europe.[6] Gather Heritage Farm wants to help change that. We are so happy to have some elderberry bushes on our farm already, and we plan to add more.

Even if you cannot grow your own elderberry bushes, you can still reap the benefits of this plant by purchasing dried elderberries from an online source. This Elderberry Syrup recipe is just one more way to help your family avoid the discomforts of seasonal colds and flu.

Elderberry Syrup

2 cups filtered water
⅔ cup dried elderberries or 1½ cups fresh
1 cup raw local honey
1 tsp. whole cloves
1 stick cinnamon
1 knob of fresh, peeled ginger

Bring the water, elderberries, and spices to a boil in a saucepan. Reduce heat, cover, and simmer on low for thirty to forty-five minutes. During the simmering, use a potato masher to crush the elderberries. Remove the saucepan from the heat.

Pour the honey into a separate glass jar. Filter the hot syrup through a sieve or cheesecloth into the honey. You might need to grab a funnel. You will want to make sure you squeeze all the liquid from the elderberries. This is why I like using a cheesecloth; I can twist it to ensure that it's completely drained out.

Stir the honey until it is dissolved in the hot syrup. Date and label the jar and store in the refrigerator. The honey acts as a natural preservative, so your syrup should be good for several months in the fridge.

When feeling under the weather, adults can take 1 teaspoon every two to four hours. Children over one year old can take ½ teaspoon every two to four hours.

Homemade echinacea tea

Echinacea is a flower also known as the purple coneflower. As the name suggests, it is usually purple, but some species may be other colors. Today more than fifty hybrids have been developed from the nine distinct species.[7]

Echinacea has been consumed for its health benefits for hundreds of years, but it has been scientifically studied only recently. Echinacea has been used throughout history as an antimicrobial to help fight infections, treat snakebites, and relieve pain. Native Americans used it to soothe coughs and sore throats.[8] Some modern studies have shown it to be effective in shortening or preventing colds and boosting the immune system.[9] Today echinacea is also used against many other infections, including the flu, urinary tract infections, vaginal yeast infections, genital herpes, bloodstream infections (septicemia), gum disease, tonsillitis, streptococcus infections, syphilis, typhoid, malaria, and diphtheria.[10]

You can use either fresh echinacea herb parts or dried parts to make echinacea tea, which is excellent for strengthening the immune system and fighting off infections, colds, and flu. There are many different kinds of echinacea tea you can make. Each starts with a basic recipe, and then additional items or essential oils are added to create healthy and beneficial variations. I want to share with you my favorite echinacea tea recipe, though I'm sure I will be developing new and fresh echinacea tea recipes for as long as my wonderful perennial echinacea plants continue growing. (And believe me, I plan to keep them growing!)

Echinacea Tea

½ cup fresh or ¼ cup dried echinacea leaves,
  roots, or flowers
8 oz. water
3½ tsp. raw honey

Simmer water in a small pot over medium heat. Add the fresh or dried echinacea. Cover and simmer for fifteen minutes. Strain tea into a mug and add honey.

NATURAL SOLUTIONS FOR ACHES, PAINS, AND MUSCLE SORENESS

All of us are going to deal with aches, pains, and muscle soreness from time to time. Sometimes our muscles get sore after we work out. Sometimes we deal with injuries, arthritic joints, or temporary problems that bring on the pain. I want to take a look at some of the natural, homemade solutions you can find to remedy these kinds of aches and pains.

Eating natural, organic, unprocessed foods is one of the best ways to ensure that you are doing all you can to get and keep your body healthy. There's something else you can do that will greatly improve the taste of your food while providing your body with healthy, powerful quantities of antioxidants and nutrients to support its systems. What is it? It's adding amazing herbs and spices that are very low in calories but dense in vitamins and minerals—like turmeric!

Turmeric is often called nature's powerhouse spice. A member of the ginger family and a main ingredient in curry, turmeric has been used as a healthy spice for thousands of years. It has proven to be very beneficial to people who are suffering from painful joints caused by arthritis. According to the *New York Times*, "a study published in *The Journal of Alternative and Complementary Medicine* in 2009 compared the active ingredient in turmeric, curcumin, with ibuprofen for pain relief in 107 people with knee osteoarthritis. The curcumin eased pain and improved function about as well as the ibuprofen."[11]

Curcumin, which gives turmeric its yellow color, has also been proven to help prevent hardening of the arteries and stop the loss of protein through the kidneys. In laboratory studies it has successfully killed cultures of some cancer cells from the skin, ovaries, and bloodstream.[12] According to WebMD, it is used to relieve "arthritis, heartburn, stomach pain, diarrhea, intestinal gas, bloating, loss of appetite, jaundice, liver problems, gallbladder disorders, headaches, bronchitis, colds, lung infections, fibromyalgia," arthritis, and joint pain.[13]

Here are some simple ways to add turmeric to your arsenal of natural health remedies to deal with those bothersome aches and pains.

Turmeric Water

To increase absorption of turmeric and get the therapeutic dose necessary for maximum benefit, add 1 tablespoon turmeric powder to a quart of boiling water, boil for ten minutes, and drink the turmeric water within six hours.[14]

Golden Turmeric Milk[15]

Golden Turmeric Milk combines the potent anti-inflammatory benefits of turmeric with the healthy, creamy base of coconut milk. You can prepare the "golden paste" ahead of time, which will allow you to quickly make a cup of golden milk whenever you would like.

For the Golden Paste

1 cup water
½ cup organic turmeric powder
1½ tsp. black pepper
5 Tbsp. virgin coconut oil

In a stainless steel pot boil the water, turmeric, and black pepper until it forms a thick paste. Continue to stir and simmer for seven to ten minutes. Remove from heat and whisk in the virgin coconut oil, being sure to fully incorporate it. Put the golden paste in a glass jar with a lid and store in the refrigerator for up to two weeks.

Once you've made your golden paste, you're ready to make the golden milk.

1 tsp. golden paste
2 cups coconut milk
⅛ tsp. vanilla (optional)
Raw honey (or stevia) to taste
Pinch of cinnamon

In a stainless steel pot slowly heat 2 cups of milk combined with 1 teaspoon of golden paste. Be sure not to let the mixture boil. Whisk to fully combine the paste with the milk. If desired, add vanilla, honey (or stevia), and cinnamon to taste.

Turmeric also has possible anti-inflammatory effects, which may be beneficial if you have low back pain. Researchers have used standardized turmeric extracts containing 400 mg to 600 mg of curcumin per tablet or capsule, taken three times a day, in studies of its effect on low back pain, according to the Palo Alto Medical Foundation. Turmeric tincture (turmeric mixed with alcohol) is typically taken three times a day in doses of 0.5 to 1.5 ml. According to LiveStrong.com, "Other suggested daily doses of turmeric include 1.5 to 3 [grams] of the cut root, 1 to 3 [grams] of dried powder root, and 30 to 90 drops of fluid extract."[16]

SOOTHING SALVES AND RUBS FOR MINOR SKIN DISCOMFORTS

When your skin is irritated or you are suffering with itching or discomfort from some bothersome condition, there are many comforting homemade rubs and salves that may bring you relief. I want to tell you about two I particularly like to make and use.

All-purpose salve

With little ones in the house, there seems to be an endless number of reasons for me to pull this salve out of the cabinet. I like to keep things very simple, which is why I really love essential oils. I have replaced so many products with essential oils and some other holistic remedies. Now my medicine shelf is very minimalistic.

This all-purpose salve is good for so many things. The coconut oil and olive oil bring nourishment, while the beeswax is known to lock in moisture and protect skin from damaging environmental factors. For children, the *best* two essential oils to have on hand are melaleuca and lavender.

Melaleuca (tea tree oil) is renowned for its cleansing and rejuvenating effect on the skin. Lavender is known as a universal oil that is extremely beneficial and helps many conditions. Combine these two together and you have a powerful weapon to aid in relief.

All-Purpose Salve

½ cup coconut oil
½ cup olive oil
⅓ cup calendula flower petals (dried)
¼ cup beeswax

15 drops melaleuca essential oil
15 drops lavender essential oil

Put the coconut oil and olive oil in a double boiler. Melt the coconut oil if it isn't melted already. Add the dried calendula flower petals and simmer on low for around two hours. Make sure to stir a few times during the process. You can also put the oil and calendula in a slow cooker and simmer on low for up to three hours. Check on it often to make sure the calendula petals are not burning.

Strain the mixture into a bowl through a cheesecloth. Then put the calendula oil back in the saucepan and add the beeswax. Melt the beeswax. Remove from heat and let cool for around fifteen minutes. Add the essential oils and stir. Pour into a glass jar and store for up to a year! Makes 1 cup.

This salve is cloth-diaper–safe and newborn-safe, as the essential oil dosages in this recipe do not exceed the recommendations for a newborn. However, if you plan to use it on a newborn, I highly recommend you use a very safe essential oil that is 100 percent pure therapeutic grade. Keep this salve on hand for *anything*.

Homemade comfrey salve

One of my favorite things about my homestead is that we have our very own comfrey patch. Of course, you don't need to grow your own comfrey to make a nourishing salve with it. There are several places online that you can purchase dried, organic comfrey leaves to make this simple homemade salve.

Comfrey has been used for medicinal purposes for more than two hundred years. Because of its allantoin content, comfrey can aid in treating wounds, swollen tissue, sores, burns, and even broken bones. When applied over inflamed tissue (bruises, sprains, or even arthritic bones), it proves to be a beneficial anti-inflammatory and pain reliever.[17]

Here is a great recipe for a soothing, homemade comfrey salve.

Comfrey Salve

½ cup coconut oil
½ cup olive oil

¼ cup beeswax
⅓ cup dried comfrey
25 drops of lavender essential oil
25 drops of melaleuca essential oil

Put the coconut oil, olive oil, and beeswax in a double boiler. Melt over medium heat. Add the comfrey and simmer on low for around two hours. Make sure to stir a few times during the process. Strain the mixture into a bowl through a cheesecloth. Let cool for a few minutes, then add the essential oils and stir. Pour into a glass or tin jars and store for up to a year! Makes 1 cup.

There are three *big* reasons to choose natural solutions for your health above traditional medicines and treatments:[18]

1. Safety—More than 200,000 people in the United States die each year from prescription medications and their often dangerous side effects. Thousands more die in hospitals as a result of medical negligence.[19]

2. Expense—Natural cures and remedies are far less expensive than the cost of doctors, medications, and insurance.

3. Effectiveness—Natural remedies work better. They treat the underlying cause, not just the symptom.

It's time for you to begin taking your own baby steps into the world of natural solutions and homemade remedies for your health concerns. Determine now that part of your journey to a naturally healthy lifestyle will include learning about the natural ways and homemade solutions you can develop for your family's use. Let's get back to nature's remedies and really start living the natural life.

Chapter 10

HOMEMADE BODY-CARE WONDERS

$\mathcal{E}$VERYDAY NATURAL LIVING is about more than just using natural, organic, homemade remedies to get rid of bothersome or irritating minor illnesses and health problems. It's also about caring for your body in such a way that you *feel wonderful, refreshed, and at peace in your own skin.* It's not only a wellness option; it's also an emotional response to the positive reactions your body is having to its newfound radiant health.

That is what I want this chapter to do for you. I want to share some homemade body-care wonders that will make you feel awesome contentment and peace. Do you think that's an impossible task? I don't! I've had all those feelings myself as I've learned to thoroughly enjoy the wonderful natural ways I can take care of my body and my family's needs.

In this section I include homemade body-care goodies you can make for yourself and your favorite adults, as well as a section of body-care recipes for children. They will all win you rave reviews. Are you ready?

WONDERFUL BATH SOAPS AND SCRUBS

For us busy adults, there is probably no more pleasurable time than the few precious moments we get to spend alone in our bathrooms, soaking in a tub of nature-enriched water or lathering on wonderful homemade lotions, soaps, shampoos, and hair conditioners. Let me pull you into that experience with a few of my favorite homemade joy-givers.

Sugar scrub bars
I already introduced you to the wonderful world of homemade sugar scrubs that will lather up and exfoliate your body in a totally

refreshing manner. My Pumpkin Scrub Bars are amazing, but there are many ways to make your own sugar scrubs.

You can make healthy sugar scrubs either as loose scrub morsels that you scoop out of a jar or make them into bars that you just grab when you are ready to step in the bath or shower. I like the bars best, but any sugar scrub beats the traditional soaps and exfoliants you can buy that are filled with questionable chemicals and additives.

It's really easy to come up with a recipe for a sugar scrub that "floats your boat." Each of us is elevated into pleasure by different smells and textures, so whatever works best for you is what you will want to use the most. Let me begin by giving you some basic ingredients to use in your homemade sugar scrubs, and then I'll suggest some of the many options you have for making your own special comfort scrub.

Basic Sugar Scrub

Put ½ to 1 cup of sugar in a bowl. You can use all white sugar, all brown sugar, a mixture of both, or even coconut sugar, sucanat, or organic cane sugar.

Add about half as much oil as sugar. You can use coconut oil, almond oil, jojoba oil, or olive oil, which are all good for use on the skin.

Next, add your favorite options to personalize your scrub. These can include essential oils, spices, pureed fruit, raw honey, or even teas. (See related sidebar for some of the most frequently used options.)

Once you have mixed your sugars, oils, and favorite additional items, put your sugar scrub into small jars. (You can also put the scrub into silicone molds and let them set in the freezer.)

Now all you have to do is step into your bath or shower and enjoy the luxurious feeling of scrubbing with your homemade sugar scrub. In the warm summer months you may want to keep your scrub in the fridge to keep the oils from liquefying. But at other times of the year, you can just let it rest right on your bathroom counter where it will entice you to use it often.

These scrubs are incredibly moisturizing, and they do a

wonderful job of getting rid of the dead cells and skin particles on your body. They can be used on the face, body, and feet, and will give you soft, silky skin. And best of all, they cost just pennies and take less than ten minutes to make.

Homemade goat milk soap

Goat's milk is packed with vitamins, minerals, natural fats, and protein. Its pH level is similar to that of humans, which makes goat's milk great for skin tolerance.[1] You can find vitamins A, B_2, C, and D in goat's milk, and many who cannot tolerate dairy find that they have no problems with goat's milk.[2]

Those who have very sensitive skin will discover that paying a few dollars more for a bar of goat soap than for conventional soap is worth it! I've had several people tell me that my soap was one of the only bars of soap that they could use without breaking out or having a skin reaction.

Soap is *not* hard to make. The soap I make is from a very basic, traditional recipe that I created using lard and lye. I also use the traditional method of cold-processing, which uses a short prep time and a long cure time. It's the easiest soap-making process, in my opinion,

Now all you have to do is step into your bath or shower and enjoy the luxurious feeling of scrubbing with your homemade sugar scrub.

SUGAR SCRUB OPTIONS

- Five to ten drops of essential oils such as peppermint, cinnamon, ginger, lavender, melaleuca, eucalyptus, lemon, frankincense, myrrh, patchouli, and sandalwood
- Spices such as cinnamon, allspice, ginger, nutmeg, pumpkin pie spice, apple pie spice, vanilla, and rosemary
- Unsweetened cocoa powder
- Raw honey
- Oatmeal
- Peach, green, or chai tea bag leaves
- Pureed cranberries, cucumber, or apple
- Zest of an orange, lemon, or grapefruit
- Tablespoon of orange, lemon, or grapefruit juice

because you are mostly waiting on the soap to cure and harden. This is the way our ancestors prepared soap, and it's the way I prefer to make my soap.

Since I use raw goat's milk, I prefer to keep the milk unheated to keep from destroying any vitamins and minerals.

You will need separate supplies to use when working with the lye. Any supplies that touch the lye should never be used on anything else. Also, this recipe is going to make an unscented bar. I have tried using essential oils and it requires way too much. However, you can add a few drops of essential oil to your bar of soap when you are washing in the shower.

If you choose to do so, there are dozens of creative soap molds you can purchase to use, but my philosophy is, who needs swirls and fun shapes? Of course, for gift-giving, you may want to investigate some of these molds. If you enjoy doing that, then by all means, go for it—but there is nothing prettier than a rustic bar of soap! Also, I make soap for my family, and most the time the kids end up making holes in the bar and pretending Spiderman can surf on it.

Homemade Goat Milk Soap

> Safety equipment—rubber gloves, long-sleeved
>   shirt, and goggles
> Digital kitchen scale*
> Immersion blender
> Soap molds or old loaf pans
> Parchment paper
> Tall stainless steel pot for melting oils
> Two thermometers*
> Glass bowls for mixing
> Rubber spatulas
> Knife to cut the soap

> Note: You can change which fats and oils you use if you would like. This is just the recipe I created and enjoy the most. I have made soap from several other recipes, but I prefer mine, as it is very moisturizing, lathers very well, and includes sustainable fats.

> 2 oz. beeswax
> 18 oz. coconut oil

5 oz. castor oil
26 oz. pastured lard
6 oz. olive oil
8.4 oz. (238.39 grams) of 100 percent pure lye
18.9 oz. frozen goat's milk (pour the measured
    goat's milk into a gallon Ziploc bag to freeze,
    and freeze the bag flat)

Collect all your supplies and block off your kitchen. I usually do this when my kids are down for a nap because of the lye.

Put parchment paper in your loaf pans to get them ready.

Measure out all the fats and oils (everything but the lye and milk) and put in a tall stainless steel pot.

Put your stove on low and slowly melt the oils and the fats. Put a thermometer in and make sure the temperature never goes above 100 degrees. Once melted, remove mixture from stove.

Take your bag of frozen goat's milk and smash it up into smaller pieces. Add it to a large glass bowl. Slowly sprinkle your lye over the frozen milk and mix with a spatula at the same time. (Make sure you are wearing your safety gear!)

Mix until the frozen milk is melted. Check the temperature of the mixture with a thermometer and do not let it go over 110 degrees. If it does, no worries, just cool it down by placing the bowl in a larger bowl filled with ice water.

Now check on your oil mixture and make sure the oils are melted and the temperature is not over 100 degrees. If it is, then cool it down by placing the bowl in ice water. You want your oil mixture and your lye mixture to be within ten degrees of each other.

Make sure you are wearing your safety gear!

Now slowly pour your lye mixture into your oil mixture. As you are pouring, put your immersion blender on low and start to mix. When all the lye mixture is added, turn your immersion blender on high and mix until you reach "trace" (this is when you can draw a line in your mixture with a spoon or spatula). It usually takes me two minutes to reach trace with this recipe, sometimes less.

Once you reach trace, you are going to need to move very quickly. Immediately, pour your mixture into your two loaf pans or your soap molds. Use your rubber spatula to clean the bowl and smooth out the top of the loaf pan.

Put the pans in a dark area out of reach of kids. Leave it alone for twenty-four hours. After around twenty-four hours, the lye will be inactive, and you will be able to touch the soap.

After twenty-four hours, remove your soap from the loaf pans and cut into individual bars. Place the bars in a dark area and let them cure for three to four weeks. I know it's torture to wait, but it's *so* worth it! After three to four weeks the bars should be ready to use.

You may want to look at my picture tutorial before you begin to make your soap.[3] But once you try it, I guarantee you will want to make more.

SOOTHING BODY BUTTERS AND RUBS

I don't need a health-oriented reason to love the feel of a luxurious homemade body butter or rub. All I need is that undeniable urge to pamper my skin with a soothing, aromatic rub. In this section I want to share some of my favorite body butters and rubs.

Body butter

I have an obsession with making body butter. There is something deeply satisfying about transforming simple ingredients into luxurious, natural, nourishing lotions. This Lavender Body Butter is a perfect example of that. It's simple to make and has only four ingredients, one of which is lavender essential oil.

Lavender essential oil has been used and cherished for centuries for its unmistakable aroma and many benefits. It is used for bathing and relaxing, and in many perfumes. Many people love its calming and relaxing effect. You can add it to your bathwater to soak away stress, or add a few drops to pillows and bedding to pro-mote a restful night's sleep. But one of my favorite ways to use lav-ender essential oil is in this recipe.

Lavender Body Butter

2 cups coconut oil
½ cup shea butter
2 Tbsp. jojoba or almond oil
25 drops of lavender essential oil*
2 Tbps. arrowroot powder (optional; some use this to cut the greasy feeling of the coconut oil)

Using a double boiler, melt the coconut oil and shea butter in a glass or stainless steel bowl over medium-low heat. Put mixture in the fridge (for around 30 minutes) or a freezer (for around 15 minutes) until the mixture becomes opaque and starts to harden along the sides. Using a stand mixer (if possible), whip the mixture until it becomes creamy, light, and fluffy.

As you are mixing, drizzle the 2 tablespoons almond or jojoba oil into the bowl. Then add the 25 drops of lavender essential oil and the arrow-root powder. Turn off mixer. Store in a glass Mason jar until you're ready to lather it all over your body!

Bonus sunscreen recipe: Add 2 tablespoons of non-nano zinc oxide and substitute beeswax for the jojoba or almond oil, and you will have a healthy sunscreen!

Sleepy-time rub

Winding down at night can be tough at times. I know my mind keeps going for minutes and sometimes hours after I lay my head down on my pillow. The same goes for our kids. Sometimes we expect that as soon as we shut their bedroom doors, they are going to be sweet little angels and fall asleep. Most of the time we are proven wrong!

Our nightly routine has become a little less rushed and a lot more pleasant.

Lately our nightly routine has become a little less rushed and a lot more pleasant. We let the kids take a long bath and get snuggled up in pajamas (we do the same), then we sit together as a family and read books. During our reading time I love to rub us all down with this Whipped Sleepy-Time Rub. I use essential oils that are known to aid in promoting a nice, restful sleep.

Whipped Sleepy-Time Rub

¼ cup cacao or cocoa butter
¼ cup coconut oil
20 drops of lavender essential oil
12 drops of vetiver essential oil*
10 drops of frankincense essential oil*
(You can substitute other essential oils that
    promote relaxation and a restful night's sleep
    such as ylang ylang, Roman chamomile,
    cedarwood, or clary sage.)

Add the cacao butter and coconut oil to a small pan and heat until melted. Remove from heat and let rest on the counter for ten minutes. Add the essential oils to the pan and then put the pan in the fridge for an hour. You want it to be firm but not too hard. Then whip it on high with an electric hand mixer until the mixture softens and forms peaks.

When your Whipped Sleepy-Time Rub is ready to use, take a pea-sized amount and massage it into your feet (and your children's feet) before bed. If desired, you can also massage it into your neck area, on your wrists, or wherever you and your family can enjoy its scent as you fall asleep. Now sleep tight!

Lip balm

I love chai tea and the way the spices in a chai tea smell. I have been making my own lip balm for years now, and I created a delicious Spiced Chai Lip Balm recipe that I know you will enjoy. We need to remember that our lips need as much pampering and moisturizing as the rest of our bodies—sometimes more.

Spiced Chai Lip Balm

1 Tbsp. coconut oil
1 Tbsp. cacao butter or raw shea butter

1 Tbsp. beeswax pastilles (or pellets)
¼ tsp. castor oil (for shine)
½ tsp. vanilla
Essential oils (4 drops cinnamon bark or cassia,
   4 drops ginger, 4 drops clove)
Small containers or old lip balm tubes that have
   been cleaned

Add the coconut oil to a small pan and heat until melted. Add the cacao or shea butter and beeswax pellets and simmer for 5–10 minutes until the butters are melted. Add the castor oil. Stir and remove from heat. Let sit until the mixture is warm to the touch but not thick. It's easier to pour into containers when it is still liquid. Add the vanilla and essential oils. Stir. Pour into your containers and enjoy! You can easily double or triple this recipe to make extras to give away to your friends!

Here's a little hint: try using your Spiced Chai Lip Balm at the very moment you are tempted to say something you might be sorry for later!

ESPECIALLY FOR THE KIDS

I like to make our nightly routine as pleasant for my kids as it is for Frank and me. Believe me when I say, if Mama isn't happy at bedtime, no one is happy! The following recipes go a long way toward making this mama happy at bedtime.

Detox bath

For everyone in our family, there's nothing like taking a hot bath. We adults may light a few candles and diffuse our favorite essential oils while we allow the troubles and duties of the day to simmer away in a soothing soak.

Our kids benefit from these bathtub times as well. I have developed a deeply comforting bath that promotes health and relaxation for them. It flushes out the toxins that have built up in their bodies and promotes sleep and relaxation. We enjoy these

> Believe me when I say, if Mama isn't happy at bedtime, no one is happy!

detox baths two to three times a week. Let me tell you how we do this.

Soothing Detox Bath

Epsom salt or magnesium flakes
Hot tub of water
Baking soda, if water is unfiltered
High-quality essential oils
Coconut oil, olive oil, or milk
Cranky, wired, and adorable kids

Add the Epsom salt to a tub of hot water.[4]

- For children under 60 pounds, add ½ cup to a standard bath.
- For children between 60 and 100 pounds, add 1 cup to a standard bath.
- For those over 100 pounds, add 2 cups or more to a standard bath.

If your water is unfiltered, add the baking soda. It helps to neutralize the chemicals in the water, especially chlorine. I have well water so I don't need to do this.

- For children under 60 pounds, add ¼ cup to a standard bath.
- For children between 60 and 100 pounds, add ½ cup to a standard bath.
- For those 100 pounds or more, add 1 cup to a standard bath.

Add the coconut oil, olive oil, or milk. It helps the essential oils bind and stick to the kids' skin, which helps to moisturize their skin. It also keeps the essential oils from sticking to the side of the tub.

- Add 1 tablespoon for kids under 60 pounds.
- Add 2 tablespoons for kids between 60 and 100 pounds.
- Add 3 tablespoons for those over 100 pounds.

Add the essential oils.

- For children under 60 pounds and over two years old, add 4 drops to a standard bath.
- For children between 60 and 100 pounds, add 6 drops to a standard bath.
- For those 100 pounds or more, add 10 drops to a standard bath.

The only thing left to add are those cranky yet adorable kids!

Here are a few additional things to keep in mind for detox bath nights.

+ Don't wash your kids' hair on these nights. The coconut oil will make their hair greasy and is hard to get out.
+ Don't use additional soaps or harsh cleansers. I recommend a mild soap such as castile soap if you must wash the kids.
+ Try to keep the kids in the bath for at least twenty minutes.

> **RELAXING ESSENTIAL OILS YOU MAY WANT TO USE**
> - Ylang ylang
> - Cedarwood
> - Frankincense
> - Eucalyptus
> - Peppermint
> - Lemon
> - Cardamom

+ Leave a glass of water beside your children's beds. Detox baths can make a person thirsty.
+ Cuddle with your kids on the couch and read a good book after they take their baths.

Homemade baby powder

Sometimes you just need a dry barrier on your little one's bum. Making homemade baby powder is so easy. Plus, the store-bought baby powders have talc in them. Breathing in talc is terrible for your lungs, and putting it on a baby's genital area is even worse.[5]

Now, now, don't go feeling all guilty on me and start thinking you are a bad mom. You are now an informed mom, so you can make the changes you need!

This recipe is simple, easy, and nourishing to your baby's bottom. It is also cloth diaper–safe.

DIY Baby Powder

¼ cup calendula flowers
¼ cup oatmeal
½ cup bentonite clay
¼ cup arrowroot powder
5 drops of therapeutic-grade lavender or
   chamomile essential oil*

Put the calendula flowers and the oatmeal in a food processor and process until it is finely ground. Add the bentonite clay and the arrowroot powder to the food processor and pulse a few times to combine. Put in a shaker bottle and apply as needed!

Let's face it—some adults might need this too!

Now, now, don't go feeling all guilty on me and start thinking you are a bad mom. You are now an informed mom, so you can make the changes you need!

This chapter has been all about pampering ourselves and our families with some wonderful homemade body-care products. Try these out and see if you don't feel just a little more refreshed and ready for the next step. And you know, you can always cuddle up with your favorite hot latte or cool drink to extend the pampered feeling. Make these items once, and you won't want to stop!

PART III

Everyday Natural Home and Garden

Chapter 11

DETOXING YOUR HOME

HE ARRIVAL OF spring every year is one of those "I love it; I hate it" times for most of us. We love the fresh, warm air and the scent of all the trees and flowers beginning to bloom again. We love opening up the windows and letting the fresh air waft into our stale, closed-up-too-long homes.

But then we remember it will soon be time to pull out the cleaning supplies and freshen up the house with some good old spring cleaning! And therein lie some of the most toxic and dangerous chemicals we will encounter. Not only are these chemicals taking a toll on our bodies, but they are also taking a toll on our home environments as well.

So let's tackle the problem of how to move to a more natural, safe way to do our spring cleaning—and extend that to any time we need to use a cleaning product in our homes.

TOP CLEANING PRODUCTS TO AVOID

I want to begin by taking a look at some of the prime chemical-laden cleaning products you should steer clear of whenever possible:[1]

+ Window or glass cleaner—These cleansers usually contain ammonia, which can irritate the eyes, skin, and respiratory system. Ammonia produces a fatal chloramine gas when it mixes with chlorinated products.

+ Conventional air fresheners—Air fresheners produce an oil film called methoxychlor in your nasal passages, which can harm the nerves in your nose over time and interfere with your ability to smell.

+ Conventional antibacterial cleaners—In addition to helping to produce new antibiotic-resistant "superbugs," antibacterial cleaners may negatively affect the immune system.[2] These cleansers also contain triclosan, which can be absorbed by the skin and cause liver damage.

+ Bleach—Bleach can burn the eyes, skin, and respiratory tract. It is a very strong corrosive and should never be mixed with ammonia products because chloramine gas fumes will be produced.

> ### HABITS FOR A CLEAN HOME[3]
>
> To avoid using harsh chemicals to clean your home, keep these simple steps in mind:
>
> - Clean spills right away.
> - Rinse stains on clothing with water immediately.
> - Clean toilet messes as soon as they happen.

+ Conventional laundry detergent—Laundry detergents contain a variety of chemicals, including phosphorus, ammonia, naphthalene, phenol, and sodium nitilotriacetate. These can cause sinus problems and various skin irritations such as rashes, itchiness, and dryness.

+ Conventional drain cleaner—Most drain cleaners contain sodium hydroxide or sulfuric acid, which can cause blindness if it gets in the eyes.

+ Conventional oven cleaner—These cleaners typically contain sodium hydroxide or potassium hydroxide, which are extremely corrosive.

+ Bleach-based cleaning powders—Cleaning powders such as Comet and Ajax contain formaldehyde (which is thought to cause cancer) and other chemicals such as benzene and chloroform. Many negative side effects can occur from these chemicals, including cancer and reproductive disorders.

+ Furniture polish—Furniture polish typically contains toxic nitrobenzene, which is easily absorbed through the skin.

+ Toilet bowl cleaners—These cleaners contain hydrochloric acid, which can corrode the skin and eyes.

+ Dishwasher detergent—These contain a highly concentrated form of dried chlorine and leave a residue every time you wash your dishes, meaning you actually consume these chemicals when you eat off these dishes.

NATURAL PRODUCTS TO USE INSTEAD OF CHEMICALS

Many of the products you already have in your home are natural, safe items you can substitute for commercial household cleansers. These common, environmentally safe products can be used alone or they can be combined to create homemade cleaning products. We'll take a look at some of my favorite DIY cleaning recipes in this chapter, but first let's look at this list of safe products you can use for your spring cleaning and year-round:[4]

+ Baking soda—cleans, deodorizes, softens water, and scours

+ Castile soap—available in liquid form, flakes, powders, or bars; biodegradable and will clean just about anything, but soaps containing petroleum distillates should be avoided

+ Lemon—one of the strongest food acids, effective against most household bacteria

+ Borax (sodium borate)—cleans, deodorizes, disinfects, and softens water; cleans wallpaper, painted walls, and floors

+ White vinegar—cuts grease and removes mildew, odors, some stains, and wax buildup

+ Washing soda—sodium carbonate decahydrate, a mineral also called SAL soda; cuts grease, removes stains, softens water, and cleans walls, tiles, sinks, and tubs; can irritate mucous membranes and should not be used on aluminum

> ## USE OF BORAX
>
> The use of borax for home-cleaning formulas where no borax is ingested has not been shown to pose health hazards. Borax is a natural substance that is noncarcinogenic and does not accumulate in the body or absorb through the skin.[5]

+ Isopropyl alcohol—an excellent disinfectant, but some recommend using ethanol or 100 proof alcohol mixed with water, as there is some indication that isopropyl alcohol buildup contributes to illness in the body

‣ Cornstarch—can be used to clean windows, polish furniture, and shampoo carpets and rugs

‣ Citrus solvent—cleans paint brushes, oil, grease, and some stains; may cause skin, lung, or eye irritations for people with multiple chemical sensitivities

EXCHANGING OLD HABITS FOR NEW ONES

The journey to everyday natural living must include taking steps to develop new, safer, more natural habits. So many of us lead busy lives, and the habits we have used to care for our homes are sometimes not the healthiest or safest. It is my recommendation that you begin your journey to a more natural home environment by simply changing a few home care habits. Here are some ideas to help you begin.

1. Change the indoor air as often as possible.

Many homes are built so airtight that little fresh air can get inside. Some of us live in cities and neighborhoods where we feel it is safer to always keep the windows closed and locked. I grew up in a home like that. My father was so cautious about keeping the windows closed so burglars couldn't get in that we had at least two locks on every window and rarely, if ever, did those windows open. A great habit to develop is to open doors and windows wide on a cold, wintry day for about five minutes. Sure, the temperature will drop for a little while, but you will be letting in some wonderful fresh air. Your walls and furnishings will retain the heat, so your home will be toasty warm again soon, and the air quality will be greatly improved. So decide to change that locked-up mind-set and open your windows from time to time.

2. Try using an essential-oil diffuser.

Aromatherapy essential-oil diffusers are small devices that send the essential-oil elements into the air. This is an excellent way to purify the air and receive the benefits of the antiseptic and antibacterial properties infused in the oils. There are many benefits to using a diffuser:

✦ They help cleanse the air. Essential oils combat microorganisms, decrease the toxicity of chemicals, and increase atmospheric oxygen.

✦ They boost the immune system. Diffusing essential oils combats seasonal distresses.

> **SEASONAL SUPPORT ESSENTIAL-OIL DIFFUSER RECIPE**
> - 2 drops lavender essential oil
> - 2 drops lemon essential oil
> - 2 drops peppermint essential oil

✦ They help you to de-stress and relax. Essential oils hit the emotional center of the brain.

✦ They help you sleep better. Essential oils are able to promote relaxation and better sleep.

✦ They set the mood. Essential oils have been used for years as mood enhancers.

3. Keep your bedrooms clean, pet-free, and food particle–free.

Don't eat in the bedroom. You spend a lot of time in the bedroom, and your times of rest and sleep should be as clean and absent of dangerous bacteria or allergens as possible. And yes, that does include picking up those dirty clothes and getting them out of the room and to the laundry daily.

4. Don't let dust and dirt build up.

I feel like the pot calling the kettle black on this one—there is rarely a time in my house when I can't find some dust someplace—but this is a necessary practice. You can get rid of dust on a regular basis by doing the following:

✦ Regularly remove clutter such as old magazines and newspapers, empty containers, junk mail, papers no longer being used, and so forth.

✦ Try insisting that all shoes stay in one place, preferably near a door where everyone comes into the house. I'm so fortunate that our farmhouse has a basement back door where everyone can drop their shoes before they come up into the house.

+ Get yourself an inexpensive feather duster and give one of your children the chore of running it over the tabletops and furniture tops once a day. It may not get all the dust out, but it will sure go a long way toward minimizing how much dust stays in your home.

+ Clean from the top down. Especially when spring cleaning, start at the top so the dust falls as you work. Clean window blinds and shelves first; wash the curtains before you scrub the floors. Dust all your decorator items, picture frames, and lamps before you vacuum the rugs. Leave scrubbing the floors for last.

Decide that one of your new habits will be to find creative ways to keep dust and dirt from accumulating. This will go a long way toward making your home clean and healthy for your family.

DECIDE TO PERMANENTLY DECLUTTER YOUR HOME

All right, I know you may wonder how the subject of decluttering can fit in a chapter about spring cleaning. But I have spent the better part of a year decluttering my home and farm, and I finally have reached a point where I feel everything is in place.

> Decide that one of your new habits will be to find creative ways to keep dust and dirt from accumulating.

I found a book and a decluttering method that has been a real eye-opener for me and inspired me to get rid of tons of stuff. This process of decluttering my home and removing things that I don't "find joy in" made my mind feel calmer and more organized. The book is *The Life-Changing Magic of Tidying Up*, and the decluttering strategy its author, Marie Kondo, developed is called the KonMari method.[6] I would highly recommend this book and this method of decluttering as one of the excellent new habits to develop as part of an everyday natural lifestyle.

I want to give you some simple suggestions I have learned from this method. They are what made me excited about the KonMari process, and I hope they will do the same for you:[7]

1. *Tidy up in the right order.* There are really only two steps to the decluttering process—discarding, and deciding where to keep things. But it is vitally important for you to discard *first.* So many people get stuck in this process by stopping the discarding by saying, "All I really have to do is find a good place to stash this thing." As soon as you do that, the work of discarding comes to a halt. When people get stuck halfway, it's usually because they start with the things that are hardest to decide whether to keep or remove.

2. *Visualize what your decluttered, tidied-up home will look like.* Years ago my mother told me the story of the woman who was given one white rose. She sat that rose on her kitchen table and immediately thought, "I can't leave it there with all those dirty dishes and things," so she proceeded to clean her kitchen table, then her stove, then her sink, and finally her entire kitchen. Then she placed that one white rose on the living room side table beside her favorite chair. The same thing happened, and she proceeded to clean up her entire living room. She continued until her entire home had been de-junked and was sparkling clean. Visualize your home without any distracting clutter. What would it look like? Be specific as you picture yourself living in a clutter-free space.

3. *Ask yourself if an item sparks joy for you.* Choose what to keep and what to throw away by holding each item in your hand and asking yourself, "Does this spark joy?" If it does, keep it. If not, get rid of it. Do this with every item in your home, including every item of clothing in your closet. Are you thrilled with the thought of being able to wear that item? If not, you don't need it.

> I am determined to pour my time and passion into what brings me the most joy and into my mission in life.

4. *Don't start with your favorite mementos.* Things that have a high sentimental value to you should be left for last. The best sequence to this is clothes first, then books, papers,

and miscellaneous items. Mementos should come last. Following that order heightens your intuitive sense of what sparks joy for you.

5. *Realize that your living space affects your body.* It is a strange phenomenon, but when you reduce what you own and essentially *detox* your house, it has a detoxing effect on your body as well. It should be a wonderful thought for you to know that tidying your house can also enhance your beauty and contribute to a healthier, trimmer body.

I am determined to pour my time and passion into what brings me the most joy and into my mission in life.

MY FAVORITE DIY CLEANING PRODUCTS

I have created some of my own favorite DIY cleaning products, and I have found some created by others that work really well in my home. I want to share a few of these DIY cleaning product recipes with you.

Natural floor cleaners

When it comes to cleaning your floors, you don't need expensive products to do the job. Essential oils are great at cleaning up the dirt while leaving a refreshing, clean aroma in the air. Cleaning your floors with essential oils is completely safe, nontoxic, frugal, and easy!

Here is a list of the best essential oils to clean your floors:

+ Protective Blend: lavender and lemon
+ Citrus Blend: lemon, lemongrass, wild orange, and lime
+ Spicy Blend: orange, clove, or cinnamon
+ Cleansing Blend: melaleuca and eucalyptus
+ Minty Refresher: peppermint and wild orange

ESSENTIAL OILS FOR SPECIFIC NEEDS

• Have ants and mice? Use peppermint.

• Feeling poopy? Use melaleuca.

• Want to disinfect? Use lemon.

There are two recipes I have developed for cleaning floors. I would recommend that you use the one that best fits your need.

Multipurpose Floor Cleaner
The beauty of using essential oils on your floors is that you don't have to worry about using a specific oil on a specific surface. Each essential oil will work on your floors. This recipe works if you have tile, hardwood, linoleum, ceramic, laminate, or vinyl. You can mix any of the oils I recommended previously to make this recipe, or you can use a single oil.

> 1 cup white vinegar
> 1 Tbsp. castile soap
> 15 drops of essential oils
> One bucket of water (approximately 5 gallons)
>
> Put all the ingredients in a bucket and use to mop the floors.

Heavy-duty floor cleaner
This is a great recipe to whip up if you have a really messy, sticky spill. Most likely, you will want to use this in your kitchen where your kids eat!

> Make the Multipurpose Floor Cleaner but add 1/4 cup baking soda. Mop the floor with the mixture. Then rinse any residue with hot water.

DIY laundry detergent

I've been making my own laundry detergent for years now. I was so scared at first to switch over to natural, homemade detergent because I had the mind-set that store-bought was best, store-bought smelled better, and store-bought would make my clothes fresher. However, when my husband and I made over our budget (I'll share more about this in chapter 16), I decided to come up with a DIY laundry detergent recipe, and it has saved us a *ton* of money. It comes out to less than seven dollars to make a batch, and each load is less than two cents. That is crazy! When you use Tide, you are spending about twelve cents a load!

3 cups borax
3 cups washing soda
3 cups baking soda
2 bars castile soap or Fels-Naptha laundry soap
30 drops of essential oil (I use a 50:50 mix
   of wild orange and lemon, but you can add
   whatever you like. The essential oils are really
   optional. I included them in this recipe because
   I just love the smell and the way essential oils
   make my clothes feel.)

Grate the soap with a cheese grater. In a large bowl, mix the borax, washing soda, and baking soda. Toss the grated soap into a food processor, then add about 1 cup of the powdered mixture from the bowl. This allows your food processor to process the soap into smaller pieces without sticking to the blades.

While the food processor is on, drop the essential oil into the mixture. This allows the essential oil to blend into the soap. Take the grated soap mixture out of the food processor and add it to the large bowl. All done!

Add 1–2 tablespoons to each load of laundry. I also add about ¼ cup of white vinegar to the load as a fabric softener. This recipe makes almost a gallon of detergent.

Furniture polish

The Eartheasy website has two great tips for making your own furniture polish. If your wood is varnished, use a glass spray bottle to combine a few drops of lemon oil with ½ cup warm water. Mix together and spray onto a soft, slightly damp cotton cloth. Wipe the furniture with the cloth then follow that up by wiping the furniture again using a dry soft cotton cloth.[8]

If your wood is unvarnished, mix 2 teaspoons of olive oil with 2

EVERYDAY NATURAL TIP

Make it one of your new habits to keep a basket where you save recycled materials you can use for your DIY recipes. Include squares of old T-shirts, glass bottles in several sizes, glass jars, bars of castile soap, boxes of baking soda, and other household items you use in your recipes, along with tools you can use when making your DIY recipes.

teaspoons of lemon juice and apply a small amount to a soft cotton cloth. Squeeze the cloth to saturate it with the mixture and apply to furniture. Use wide strokes to distribute the oil evenly.[9]

Natural glass cleaner

It is very easy to make your own homemade glass cleaner, and the benefits of doing so are long lasting. You will be able to get dangerous toxins out of your home and life by getting rid of the popular but chemical-laden glass cleaners on the market. You will clean up your environment by creating a toxin-free homemade glass cleaner, and you will save money.

It's likely that your mother and/or grandmother used simple vinegar to clean her mirrors and glass, perhaps even applying it with some crumpled up newspaper. It worked well but probably left a few streaks.

> Now you really are living an everyday natural lifestyle, and it is affecting even the environment of your home.

I like using an empty glass spray bottle to hold my homemade glass cleaner. I like to partially fill the glass spray bottle with filtered water, and add 2–3 tablespoons of white vinegar, about 2 drops wild orange essential oil, and 6–8 drops of lemon essential oil. Then I add more water until the bottle is full. My glass cleaner is ready to go. I just shake well before using each time.

Natural multipurpose citrus cleaner[10]

This is a super easy and effective cleaner to use on your kitchen counters, sink, stove, table, and in your bathroom.

Orange peels (or other citrus peels)
1 Tbsp. salt
White vinegar
Distilled water
5–10 drops of your favorite essential oils

Cut your orange peels and fill an empty glass container. Add some salt to the orange peels and let them sit twenty to thirty minutes. This will pull the oils from the peels and make your cleaning solution stronger. Fill the container with a 50:50 mixture of distilled water and white vinegar. Cover with a tight-fitting lid and let the solution sit for two to three weeks. The longer it

sits, the better. Strain the solution and fill a recycled glass spray bottle with your natural orange
cleaner. Add any essential oils you want to use
at this time.

This will become a cleaner you love and use frequently. You won't
be breathing in any awful fumes as you work, and it is super cheap
to make. You will want to start a new solution as soon as you start
using yours so you have it ready when you run out.

LEARN TO LOVE SPRING CLEANING

What a wonderful feeling to know that you have thoroughly dis-
posed of all the dirt, clutter, stale air, toxic chemicals, and dangerous
solutions that used to be a part of your so-called spring cleaning
adventure. Now you really are living an everyday natural lifestyle,
and it is affecting even the environment of your home.

Once you finish initiating these new healthy habits in your home,
sit back and bask in the glory of a natural, fresh, safe home. This
new way of life is sure to give you a lot of joy and set your family on
a path to a healthier life.

Chapter 12

GARDENING LIKE THE MASTER GARDENER

I SPENT SOME TIME in chapter 4 discussing tips to help you begin to grow some of your own food. We looked at some options for container growing, and I even included some ideas for starting a small backyard garden plot to grow a few veggies.

In this chapter we are going to take an expansive look at the whole idea of raising your own vegetables and fruit by having a garden that supplies the majority of the foods for your healthy everyday natural menus. As we begin this chapter, think with me for a moment about that first luscious garden designed by our Creator. He knew just what to plant, where to plant it, and how to make it grow. How can we learn to garden like the master gardener? Let's examine three aspects of this subject of natural gardening:

- How to plan and plant your organic, natural vegetable garden
- How to have a natural garden without using chemical pesticides
- How to harvest and preserve your organic vegetables for use in your family's menus

Organic gardening is the way our great-grandparents gardened, the way food was raised for hundreds of years before chemical pesticides and synthetic fertilizers appeared on the scene. Today more and more people want to take a more active role in supplying their families with healthy, pesticide- and chemical-free food.

At Gather Heritage Farm we have chosen to concentrate on growing tomorrow from the heritage of yesterday. We are choosing heritage breeds (rare livestock breeds) for our homestead menagerie and filling our gardens with heritage and heirloom plants. My husband and I understand the importance of heritage—because we are the beneficiaries of a rich legacy.

Martin and Mary Kidder, my ancestors who lived during the 1800s, also raised plants and animals on a farm probably much like ours. I have Mary Kidder's diary from 1879, and I draw inspiration from the record of how she lived her life. Farming was hard then, probably much harder than anything I will have to face. On one particularly busy day she wrote:

> Martin gone down to ditching and I have been into almost everything. Cleaning house. Taking care of butter. Doing all the chores both outdoors and indoors. Making tomato preserves, and last—but not least—drawing water out of the well. It was not no little chore either, but done. But O my how my back aches. Good-bye, I am going to bed.

There have already been nights when I felt exactly like that—my back ached, but my chores were done and all I wanted to do was to crawl into bed. But her heritage to me is much more valuable than identifying with her aching back.

So for us, the Ritz family of Gather Heritage Farm, raising heritage plants and animals allows us to help preserve essential genetic traits—self-sufficiency, foraging ability, and maternal instincts in our animals, and resistance to diseases and parasites among our plants. Heritage breeds store a wealth of genetic resources that are important for tomorrow; heritage animals and plants are the seed of yesterday that will build a better tomorrow.

HOW TO PLAN AND PLANT YOUR ORGANIC GARDEN

If you want to grow an organic garden, you can't just pick up your shovel and a packet of seeds, stick them in the ground somewhere, and expect to be successful. Knowledge is the key to productive gardening.

Our dream farm came with ready-made flower and vegetable gardens. What a blessing for us! The former owner was a master gardener, and it's going to take me some time to get a grip on how to manage what has already been planted. But I'm determined to grow into a mini-master gardener as soon as possible. For now I want to share a few secrets I've found from my beginning research into gardening.

I think there are four important questions to answer for yourself before you pick up that shovel and seed packet.

1. What do you need in order to plant your garden?

In chapter 4 I explained how anyone can plant garden plants,

> What you grow will be partially determined by how much space you have available.

even if you live in an urban apartment with only a tiny cement patio. But here we are talking about having a larger organic garden that can supply a good portion of your family's vegetable needs. When you are considering where to begin, there are some crucial things you must think about and do to ensure that your garden produces a healthy harvest.

- *Consider the time and effort needed to maintain your garden.* Do the necessary research to learn all you can about organic gardening and then draw up a weekly checklist of maintenance tasks you will need to complete. If you want to be successful at gardening, you will need to stick to it.

- *Consider the light requirements for your plants.* "Full sun" means six or more hours of direct sunlight, and "some (or partial) shade" means that those plants don't want to be wilting in the sun all day long.

- *Consider the needs of your soil.* This is your most important starting task. Take a sample of your soil to your local university extension office for testing to determine what nutrients you need to add, or do it yourself using a store-bought soil sample test. Good soil has the right combination of silt, clay, and organic material. If your soil is sandy, you will need to work in a higher ratio of organic material to a depth of at least four to six inches. If you have clay soil, you will need to add compost material to it.

- *Don't overdose your soil with added nutrients.* Even the fertilizer made for organic gardening comes with specific instructions that must be followed to the letter for best results. I like to use natural methods to eliminate garden pests, which we will discuss later in this chapter.

+ *Don't overwater or underwater your garden.* It is recommended that you stick your finger about an inch into the soil, and if it feels dry, water thoroughly. If the soil is still moist, wait a day and check again. Avoid watering above the plants, as it can cause leaf spot and blight problems. Water directly over the plant's roots.

2. What are you going to plant in your garden?

When you are deciding what to plant, start small. Don't plant more than your family will eat and end up wasting food or feeling overwhelmed, thinking gardening is just too hard. Think about how much your family needs, and keep in mind that vegetables such as tomatoes, peppers, and squash provide continuously throughout the season, so you only need to plant as much as you will actually consume. Other vegetables such as carrots, radishes, and corn produce annually, so you will want to plant more of these crops if your family enjoys having them often. Do some research online and see what others are recommending as the most important vegetables to grow.[1]

Of course, what you grow will be partially determined by how much space you have available. Remember that you don't need a large space. You can have a good harvest from just a few container plants.

3. When are you going to plant your garden?

Starting seeds indoors can help you get a jump-start on spring. Do your research and learn what you need and get tips for successful seed starting before you begin!

+ The right time to plant your seedlings outside in your garden depends on where you live. For example, summertime gardening can be a challenge with the hot, humid summers and mild winters in the South. Heat-tolerant plants will do best. *The Old Farmer's Almanac* (www .almanac.com) has a seed-planting calculator on its website that can help you determine the best seed-starting dates for your area.

+ Vegetable gardening is divided into climate groups: cool season and warm season. To ensure that you choose the right crops for your area, remember:

1. Plant for your zone.[2] The US Department of Agriculture has developed a Hardiness Zone map, which can help you choose plants that will thrive in your area.

2. Cool season vegetables germinate best in cool soil. They are usually planted just as soon as the soil can be worked in the spring.

3. Warm season crops can be started indoors, but wait until at least two weeks after the average frost date for your region to plant outdoors. Give them some shade while they adjust to outdoor temperatures.

Growing your own food can be a rewarding adventure. There's nothing like picking the vegetables you planted and serving them to your family the very same day. Food doesn't get any fresher than that![3]

4. When will you be able to enjoy the harvest from your garden?
During the time between planting and harvest you need to diligently care for your plants. Your veggies will grow faster and better if you feed them properly with only natural products. If you have plant-eating livestock, your own compost pile of their manure would make a great source of fertilizer for your plants. Another option is to buy prepackaged organic material online or at your garden store.[4] Here are a few other things to keep in mind:

+ It is a good idea to build your own compost station. Creating a compost station that is rich in minerals doesn't take much effort. Throw in fruit and veggie scraps, used tea bags and coffee grounds (the filters too), egg shells, and even dog hair. A good quality compost will enrich your soil and give your plants much-needed nutrients.[5]

+ Plan how you will store and use your harvest well in advance. If you don't, your abundant harvest will overwhelm you. Each day pick what is ripe, because that will encourage your plants to grow more. Remember, most vegetables are at their most tender and have the most flavor when they're still relatively small. For instance, zucchini are best at six or seven inches long; after that point, they become tough.[6]

+ Track what you have planted. Because there are so many vegetable varieties, you could lose track of the size and characteristics each was designed to display. So you may want to use the seed packet so you know what to expect from your crops. For instance, if you plant a watermelon variety that ripens at eight inches across, it will take less time for it to reach its prime than one intended to weigh twenty-five pounds.[7]

+ At harvest time watch for problems (these include yellowing leaves or rotting fruit) and remove the problem areas. Prune the plant so it produces fruit you can actually eat.[8]

If you do the proper research and learn the lessons mentioned here, who knows? You may become the master gardener you always dreamed of being.

NATURAL REMEDIES FOR GARDEN PESTS

One thing that can discourage a new organic gardener faster than anything else is the abundance of garden pests that want to take over your veggies and prevent you from getting your first good harvest. It's tempting to buy the latest pesticide that promises to rid your garden of those unwanted creepy-crawlies, but that would defeat your purpose. So here are a few natural options for pest control:

+ *Diatomaceous earth*—"a soft, crumbly, porous sedimentary deposit formed from the fossil remains of diatoms"; effective against a variety of pests[9]

+ *Plant collars*—prevent slugs and other pests from getting on the plant

+ *Borax and sugar*—used to kill ants around the base of the plant

+ *Row covers*—a garden fabric or netting that is used to cover young plants

+ *Natural dishwashing liquid*—used to make homemade pest spray

- *BT spray*—an organic formula that kills insects and larvae
- *Dipel dust*—used by commercial organic growers to control insects on vegetables
- *Japanese beetle traps*—these use a pheromone to lure beetles and then traps them
- *Spinosad*—"a natural substance made by a soil bacterium that can be toxic to insects";[10] typically available as an organic insect spray
- *Essential oils*—rosemary, melaleuca, peppermint, and thyme are just a few essential oils that can help keep away garden insects

Organic gardeners are familiar with some common pests that like to attack plants. A recent survey of organic gardeners identified the twelve most bothersome garden insects, and fortunately there are natural ways to control each of them:[11]

1. *Slugs*—Gardeners frequently complain that these slimy critters cause trouble year after year. One gardening expert shared several other gardeners' tips for dealing with slugs. These experts mentioned a variety of natural ways to eliminate slugs from gardens, including letting garden critters such as chickens and chipmunks eat them, setting out partially consumed beer bottles so they can drown in the beer, spreading crushed eggshells, spraying salt water or homemade garden soap, handpicking, and spreading copper around the perimeter.[12]

2. *Squash bugs*—Squash bugs frequently sabotage summer and winter squash harvests. *The Free Range Life* gardening blog shares six ways to control squash bugs.[13] These include handpicking, planting companion plants (plants grown together for the benefit of each plant), attracting beneficial insects, using diatomaceous earth, watching your mulch, and overplanting your squash. You will find more information on *The Free Range Life* website (www.thefreerangelife.com).

3. *Aphids*—These little pests have tried to take over many a garden. However, several home gardeners have developed effective warfare methods, which include pruning, applying

insecticidal soap, attracting beneficial insects, and planting companion plants. The Gardening Know How website (www.gardeningknowhow.com) gives detailed information about how to get rid of aphids naturally.[14]

4. *Imported cabbage worms*—Experienced gardeners recommend that if you see little white butterflies in your garden, you need to take action to protect your plants before these cabbage worm moths lay eggs. There are several ways to control them naturally, including attracting paper wasps and yellow jackets, which will eat cabbage worms. Other gardeners recommend biological pesticides but report that companion planting and garlic-pepper sprays had disappointing results. One experienced gardener shared seven natural ways to get rid of these nasty pests.[15]

5. *Squash vine borers*—These vine borers cause trouble for many gardeners. Most gardeners recommend that the best control methods are crop rotation and growing resistant squash varieties. The Toxic Free NC website (toxicfreenc.org) gives wonderful recommendations for dealing with these garden enemies.

NATURAL INSECTICIDE FOR SOFT-BODIED PESTS

Thanks to blogger Marie Stegner for sharing a recipe for an effective insecticide that works on soft-bodied pests but won't harm your plants. Put several cloves of crushed garlic, 1/4 cup canola oil, 3 tablespoons hot pepper sauce, and 1/2 teaspoon liquid soap in 1 gallon of water. Mix well. Put into a spray bottle and shake well before each use.[16]

6. *Japanese beetles*—Although Japanese beetles are not a big problem in extremely hot or cold climates, they came in sixth in the Mother Earth News survey of the top twelve most troublesome pests for gardeners. There are several effective ways to get rid of Japanese beetles, including handpicking and planting companion plants, but things like garlic-pepper spray and row covers had high failure rates. Many home gardeners enlist the help of guinea fowl and ducks as well as springtime bug-eating birds. The experienced

gardeners at VeggieGardener.com share several natural ways to control these garden enemies.

7. *Tomato hornworms*—Forty-two percent of gardeners surveyed battled infestations of tomato hornworms. Many gardeners preferred handpicking because these pests are large and easy to spot. Gardeners also recommend using wasps and companion plants for reducing their hornworm problems. VeggieGardener.com knows these nuisance caterpillars can destroy a plant in no time—they are eating machines. This website gives several tips for finding and eliminating these pests in each stage of their life.[17]

8. *Cutworms*—Although many gardeners report problems with cutworms, most recommend the common practice of placing rigid collars (made from drinking cups or tissue rolls) around seedling stems to protect them. One gardener with ten years' experience said he had never encountered this pest until he became a Montana homesteader.

> ### MAKE YOUR OWN NATURAL PESTICIDE
>
> You can make a natural pesticide using your blender. (This recipe is, again, thanks to blogger Marie Stegner.) Puree 4 onions, 2 garlic cloves, 2 tablespoons cayenne pepper, and 1 quart of water in your blender. Set aside and dilute two tablespoons soap flakes in 2 gallons of water. Add the contents of the blender to the diluted soap flakes. Stir or shake well and divide into several glass spray bottles. Use as needed.[18]

However, he learned that cutworms can quickly decimate your garden. You can read the research and tips he discovered for dealing with these garden enemies at www .montanahomesteader.com.[19]

9. *Grasshoppers*—Grasshoppers have been a problem for gardeners since biblical times, but many gardeners say the problem seems to be getting worse. Some experienced gardeners mentioned an interesting repellant using chickens. They suggested constructing a chicken moat around the fenced garden perimeter. This is a strip of dry land enclosed by a fence that surrounds a garden. Chicken

are allowed to roam the "moat" by day, eating the various pests that might try to invade the garden.[20]

10. *Cucumber beetles*—The danger with these pests is the fact that they transmit deadly bacterial wilt to cucumbers and melons. Some effective treatments include handpicking, good garden cleanup of plant debris, and row covers. Some gardeners have found success with companion planting and setting out yellow sticky traps. The Gardening Knowhow website has some thorough information about identifying and controlling cucumber beetles.[21]

11. *Corn earworms*—These were listed as serious pests by many of the gardeners surveyed, and the variety of methods for eliminating them included adding a few drops of oil to the tips of the ears, choosing pest-resistant corn varieties, and popping off the end of the ear to remove the damage from earworms. The Planet Natural website gives a great description of these garden pests, discusses the damage they do to corn, and describes several natural ways to control corn earworms.[22]

12. *Whitefly problems*—These tiny pests have caused gardeners a great deal of frustration. These common insects have developed resistance to many synthetic pesticides, but there are proven organic techniques for eliminating them, including putting down yellow sticky traps (a sticky paper created for that use, much like the old flypaper your grandmother probably used), using the Bug Blaster (which sprays full pressure water into the center of plants where insects hide without harming the plants), releasing natural predators such as ladybugs and lacewing larvae to feed on their eggs, and spraying organic or homemade pesticides and insecticidal soaps.[23]

Let's get busy driving off these pests!

Now that you've read through this list of the twelve most troublesome garden pests, you are probably hoping—*just as I am*—that none, or at least only one or two, of these insects will find their way into your garden. Remember, you may lose a battle or two with some of these garden pests. But if you arm yourself with this information and have ready the weapons to get rid of these enemies, you can win the war and reap a wonderful harvest from your garden. Let's get busy driving off these pests!

HARVESTING AND PRESERVING YOUR ORGANIC VEGETABLES

After all your hard work protecting your garden, you'll be ready to enjoy the fruit of your labor. In this section I want to get you excited about a great way you can ensure that your harvested garden vegetables and fruits will stay available for you to feast on between each harvest. I want to give you some information about root cellars.

People have used root cellars for hundreds of years. They have one purpose— to provide you with long-term storage for your harvested fruits and vegetables. Underground storage facilities from the Iron Age have been discovered, and the early North American colonists knew how to preserve their crops from watching their parents and grandparents garden.

> ### EVERYDAY NATURAL GARDENING TIP
>
> You can save money on your next garden by saving seeds. It's already a great feeling to not have to depend on anyone else for the food your serve your family. Seed saving is just another step toward being food self-sufficient.[24]

Many of my ancestors were farmers, and each generation used some kind of root cellar to store their harvest during the winter. Before refrigeration, the root cellar was essential in order to keep turnips, carrots, potatoes, beets, parsnips, and other root vegetables fresh through the winter months. My mother grew up in Michigan and remembers vividly the root cellar in her basement, built by her father right next to the playhouse he built for my mother and her sister. It was my mother's job to get potatoes out of the potato bin and bring up various Mason jars stored there by her mother, who was an avid canner.

The root cellar is making a comeback among homesteaders and natural living advocates who want to reduce expenses by growing and storing their own produce. I'm doing my best to learn how to maximize its usage, and I want to share some of this information with you so you can consider doing the same thing.

Root cellar basics

There are three basic conditions a root cellar should meet. The closer you come to matching these ideal conditions in your vegetable storage area, the better your produce will keep:[25]

1. *Humidity*—High humidity is essential. Most root crops and leafy veggies keep best in humidity of 90 to 95 percent. There are three ways to maintain this level of humidity: install a dirt floor and add water when needed by setting out pans of water; place damp burlap over the produce; or pack the veggies in damp sawdust, sand, or moss.

2. *Ventilation*—Air needs to be circulated through your root cellar. Because warm air rises and cool air falls, put the air intake (where the air enters) down low and the outlet (where it exits, possibly a window) up high.

3. *Temperature*—This is the most important thing. You can borrow cold from the ground or by letting cold night air into the cellar.

Twenty-two foods you can store in a root cellar

Your root cellar will work for you as long as you pay close attention to the crop varieties you choose, when you harvest your crops, and whether you are using the best storage conditions for each type of fruit or vegetable. Contact your cooperative extension office, an educational resource formed in partnership with the National Institute of Food and Agriculture, for advice on specific storage varieties for your region. Here is a list of twenty-two crop varieties you may choose to store.[26]

Cold and damp storage

Store these at 32 to 40 degrees Fahrenheit with 90 to 95 percent humidity. Research each of these items to determine when to harvest and how to store them.

1. Apples
2. Beets
3. Broccoli
4. Brussels sprouts
5. Cabbage
6. Carrots
7. Jerusalem artichokes
8. Leeks
9. Parsnips
10. Pears
11. Potatoes
12. Rutabagas
13. Turnips
14. Winter radishes

Cool and dry storage
Store these varieties at 50 to 60 degrees Fahrenheit, with 60 to 70 percent humidity.

15. Beans (dried)
16. Garlic
17. Onions
18. Pumpkins
19. Squash
20. Sweet potatoes
21. Tomatillos
22. Tomatoes

According to Mother Earth News, having your own root cellar will "make it possible for you to enjoy fresh endive in December; tender, savory Chinese cabbage in January; juicy apples in February; crisp carrots in March; and sturdy, unsprayed potatoes in April—all without boiling a jar, blanching a vegetable, or filling a freezer bag."[27]

A root cellar will save time, money, and supplies. Your utility bills will be lower because you are not heating large kettles of water for canning. You won't have to stuff so much into the freezer, and you won't need to buy new jar lids or freezer bags.[28]

By planning ahead, you can plant enough crops to give you extra to preserve in your root cellar. You and your family and friends will not only have delicious, fresh fruits and vegetables during the growing season, but you will also be able to enjoy your bumper crop during the cold winter months through the wonderful benefits of root cellaring. If you follow some of the simple procedures for gardening that I've given you in this chapter, you will develop your own gardening expertise and will have wonderful, fresh produce. You will truly be able to garden like our Creator, the master gardener.

Everyday Natural Farm

Chapter 13

RAISING LIVESTOCK NATURALLY

*A*s I HAVE mentioned several times in this book, on our Gather Heritage Farm we have chosen to concentrate on growing heritage breeds (rare livestock breeds) for our homestead menagerie. Heritage breeds store a wealth of genetic resources that are important for tomorrow—heritage animals and plants are the seed of yesterday that will build a better tomorrow.

By raising heritage breeds we can also ensure that we are giving our animals only the very best foods and providing the safest, most pollutant-free pasture for them to feed from. Our chickens, ducks, geese, and turkey run around freely on healthy, grassy pastures and receive supplemental feed that is free of GMOs, antibiotics, and processing by-products. We refuse to use chemical pesticides either in their food or in their bodies. I've learned that there are countless ways to use essential oils around our farm and even directly on our animals. We also mix up grain-free, corn-free, and soy-free feeds for them.

I know that not everyone is able to own a farm where many different animals are raised. However, I believe it is very possible for many people to homestead with a few animals, maybe some chickens and goats or perhaps rabbits and chickens. For that reason, I want to share some natural tips to keep in mind when raising any kind of animals or poultry. My hope is that this chapter will embolden you to take those first scary steps toward establishing your own natural homestead with a few animals to help meet your food needs.

RAISING CHICKENS AND OTHER POULTRY

Some people have eaten chicken that was raised on a farm, and know what it's like to raise and butcher poultry. But many people today get their chickens from the grocery store, not the farm, so they're not aware of exactly how their poultry is raised or butchered.

Sometimes ignorance is bliss. Chickens today are raised very differently from the way they were in the "old days." Supermarket chickens are raised in terrible conditions. Most never get to see the light of day and are sometimes butchered at only four or five weeks old. They are stuffed in overcrowded quarters, and their beaks have been cut off so the stress of living with thousands of other birds doesn't cause them to peck their fellows to death.[1]

> I want this chapter to embolden you to take those first scary steps toward establishing your own natural homestead with a few animals to help meet your food needs.

It is for these reasons, and because we want to be sure the food we eat is as organic and free of pesticides and chemicals as possible, that we raise both egg-laying hens and chickens for meat. In this section we'll look at how to raise pastured meat chickens, which are called *broilers* in most instances.

If you want to attempt to raise poultry for your family, make sure you do your own research before you begin. Then put a plan together that includes answers to these questions:[2]

+ Will you use a pen or day-range production system?
+ How many birds will you raise the first year?
+ Who will do the work?
+ When do you want your first chicks to arrive?
+ Who will process the broilers?
+ Where and how will you market the birds?

You will also need to decide what kind of meat chickens you will raise. The kind of meat chicken that is most widely produced is the Cornish Cross, which is a bird that grows so fast that sometimes its heart explodes and its legs give out because it can't support its unnatural weight. A slower growing chicken is the Freedom Ranger, which is a hybrid breed (a cross between a commercial and a heritage breed) and has fewer problems than the Cornish Cross. You may even choose to stick with the older standard breeds like the Delaware or Barred Rock, which are also laying birds.

You will need the following equipment:

1. *Brooding lamp*—This is a 250-watt red light in a reflective housing that provides heat for the chicks that don't yet have feathers to keep them warm. The Brinsea EcoGlow chick brooder uses less power and is much safer than a traditional bulb.

2. *Thermometer*—The best thermometers are those used to monitor food temperatures. They have a probe on a wire attached to a separate base.

3. *Bedding*—The bedding on the coop floor is often made of pine shavings and will provide a soft place for the chicks to walk and will also absorb droppings. Paper towels placed on top of the pine shavings work great for a few days because they help to prevent the chicks from eating the shavings. After a few days, switch to just the pine shavings, a few inches thick. Pine is recommended. Cedar is toxic to poultry. Make sure there are enough shavings to keep the chicks dry. Put fresh shavings down each day or consider the deep litter method of adding fresh shavings to the top every day.

4. *Feeders and waterers*—You will likely be feeding a number of chicks, and you won't want them to run out of feed or water. A feeder such as the Little Giant Eleven-Pounds Plastic Hanging Poultry Feeder will keep you from running out. You have a couple of choices for waterers. The Chicken Water Nipples device is cheap and easy to hook up. Or you may want something movable like the 5 Gallon Chicken Waterer. Just be sure to give the base a good rinse once in a while.

> **YOUR CHICKEN COOP**
>
> There are a couple of different types and features to consider. A chicken coop with a run is a more permanent design. It includes a fenced-in area outside where the chickens can run around and a sheltered space inside the coop. You can find several different designs online.

Processing your meat chickens

Butchering your own chickens is not for the faint of heart. You need to kill them quickly, dunk them in hot water, get their feathers off, gut them, and package them. If you are planning to process your own chickens for meat, you will find complete instructions online in an article titled "How to Process Chickens."[3] An easier way is to take them to a processor or butcher shop. You will be eating this food, so do your research on the butcher. Talk to them about costs and packaging. Most will vacuum seal the birds at a cost per bird.

There is an emotional component to raising chickens. We raise them from babies, laugh at their antics, and work hard to give them a good life with nutritious food and a comfortable home. Then it comes time to kill them. We choose to treat all living things with respect and thank them for providing food for us. That doesn't mean there isn't some sadness, but overall this works best for us.

Caring for other poultry

The methods and tips I included previously for meat chickens will be pretty much the same for raising other poultry such as ducks, turkeys, or geese. We raise all these on Gather Heritage Farm, and I would recommend that you do careful research before you begin raising other poultry. Here are some tips to keep in mind when raising other types of poultry.

Turkeys

If you are hoping to save money by raising your Thanksgiving turkey yourself, that plan likely won't work out. It will be hard to compete with the sale price of the commercially grown supermarket turkeys.

You will be challenged to keep your turkey free from predators. Just about every wild critter (and even some domesticated ones) is on the prowl for a big, juicy turkey meal.

> There is an emotional component to raising chickens.

Turkeys have really cute personalities and love to be around people. It may be hard to decide if they are your family pet or your Thanksgiving Day meal.

If you have a large, lush pasture, your turkeys can be free-range, moving from area to area as they deplete the grasses and eat the bugs.

If you have a smaller pasture, you may want to consider whether you can provide enough food material for the birds to thrive. For pastured or limited-range turkeys, alfalfa, clover, and grasses such as orchard grass serve turkeys very well; however, the tall fescue grass is not recommended because it chokes out other plants and is hard for turkeys to move through.

Ducks

There are five basic things that you need to be aware of before you begin raising ducks:

1. Your ducklings need specialized brooding time.
2. Your mature ducks need ample, relatively clean water to drink and bathe in.
3. Ducks need a combination of forage and balanced feed to eat.
4. Ducks need shelter and protection from predators.
5. You need to keep your ducks in good health.

Take good care of your flock, and they will thank you daily in their own cheerful, quacking, tail-wagging duck fashion. Many people believe ducks to be the happiest animals in the barnyard!

Geese

Geese are inexpensive and perhaps the easiest to raise of all poultry. They are extremely hardy and are rarely affected by disease or insects. From an age of just two weeks, they begin to gain roughly a pound a week until they are about twelve weeks old if they are given plenty of water and grass. They can be eaten at twelve weeks old, and when this happens they are called "green geese."[4]

Geese don't need much. A simple shed to provide shelter from the weather is all they need; mostly they like to roam around in the open, even at night. As for fencing, any low wall or fence that is at least thirty-six inches high will hold them. When it is time for them to breed, geese make their own nests and hatch their own eggs.[5]

> Take good care of your flock and they will thank you daily in their own cheerful, quacking, tail-wagging duck fashion.

The American Buff geese, unlike other breeds, are very calm, have a wonderful disposition, and take great care of their goslings— qualities I find important in animals and humans alike. Very smart, friendly, and affectionate, the breed is well-suited for the average home.[6]

RAISING GOATS

If you have followed me for a while, you already know that my entire family loved raising dairy goats when we had less land. When we moved into our ten-acre farm, we decided we had enough room for a milk cow, so we sold our goat herd. However, we raised dairy goats for about four years, so I'm excited to share with you how to raise these wonderful animals. I guarantee you will enjoy them!

Regardless of whether you have one acre (we got our first goats when we lived on three rented acres) or hundreds, whether your land is sloping or flat, completely forested or filled with green pasture land, you can raise dairy goats for milk. Just two dairy goats will give you an average of one to two gallons of milk a day for ten months and keep your family stocked with wonderful raw dairy goat milk all year. You will also have milk for making cheese, yogurt, and even ice cream.

Goats are hardy and adapt well to changing climates. They forage and graze, need little space, and are not very expensive to keep. But best of all, they are highly intelligent and very friendly. Because they are extremely curious and agile, their antics can keep you laughing for hours.

What kinds of goats are the best to raise?

We had a mixed herd of Alpines and Nubians. Alpines give a ton of milk, which is why we chose that breed. Nubians are probably the most adorable goats I have ever seen. We love their personality, and their milk is definitely higher in butterfat, making it a great resource for cheese making.

It is very important that you purchase your dairy goats from a reputable dairy goat breeder and that you start with healthy stock

EVERYDAY NATURAL
FARM TIP

Goat manure and bedding make great fertilizer for the garden.[7]

that has been tested for CAE (caprine arthritis encephalitis, a virus that can cause encephalitis in children and chronic joint disease in adults) with proven genetics.

What kind of shelter do goats need?

Your dairy goats will need some kind of shelter. It doesn't have to be fancy—anything from an old building to a small shed will do—but it does have to be clean, dry, and well-ventilated. Experts recommend at least fifteen square feet of housing per goat. Stalls should have a rack for hay, a trough or some kind of box for grain, and a holder for a water pail. Leave some extra space to store feed and other supplies, and a milking stand. Keep the goats' bedding clean and dry.[8]

Goats will need plenty of outside space to run around and forage. The pasture should be at least two hundred square feet, and more is more. Also keep in mind that free-range goats need sturdy fending. They will try to escape—and are pretty good at it. They can squeeze through small spaces, hop over fences, and break out of weakly secured areas.[9]

Don't be a cautionary tale. Make sure your fencing is at least four feet high.[10] We have used galvanized fencing wire that is about four feet high and no electric fence, and it worked perfectly. We now have strung electrified wire along the top of our wire fencing because the previous owners of our house had a smaller breed of goats and didn't make their fencing four feet tall. Our larger dairy goats were able to jump right over it and make their way over to my beautiful orchard for a snack. Goats do *not* like getting shocked by an electric fence and will avoid it like the plague!

What should goats eat?

It's really best to let your goats forage in the pasture for 90 to 100 percent of their food intake. Be aware that some plants, such as oleander and wild onions, are poisonous to goats. If you don't have pasture and forage available, then you will need to supply quality hay for them at all times.

In addition to pasture and forage (hay and silage), we gave our milking female goats (called "does") some extra grain every day to supply extra protein (12 to 16 percent more) and give their milk supply a small boost. Grain was only given to our pregnant does and to our milking does when we were milking them. They got about one cup of our homemade grain for each quart of milk they were giving us. We have always left the goat kids with their mothers, so if they are feeding their babies and giving us milk, we give them a little more than one cup of grain per quart of milk we are getting. We also add a scoop of alfalfa pellets or Chaffhaye (bagged forage made with alfalfa) to the feeder when we are milking the goats. We also provide our goats with fresh water at all times.

Deciding to raise dairy goats was one of the best homesteading decisions we have made; the goat was our gateway homestead animal. Our goats became a part of our family, and I can just about guarantee that you will feel the same way if you try raising goats.

RAISING BEEF CATTLE

We recently added two Irish Dexter cows to our barnyard menagerie. Both are steers we are raising for meat. There are some very practical reasons to choose to raise Dexter cattle. Raising a Dexter cow has been compared to eating potato chips—it's almost impossible to settle for just one!

Raising grass-fed beef cattle takes a lot of work, but it often produces great results. If you have ever compared the taste of grass-fed, mature beef to conventionally raised supermarket beef, then you know exactly how delicious grass-fed beef is.

Pros and cons of raising cattle

Like with any homesteading venture, there are pros and cons to raising cattle. Here are a few to consider as you start:[11]

Cons

+ *Space*—Depending on your climate, a good rule of thumb is to have an acre per cow.
+ *Cost of hay*—Even if you have lots of land for grazing, your cows will need feed in the winter months. The hay bill for a herd of six cattle will be around nine hundred dollars for the year, depending on the going rate.
+ *Fencing*—You should investigate both barbed wire fencing and electric fencing and decide which option will work best for you. Remember that cattle are notorious for

getting out of fencing of all kinds. You'll need to stay ready to herd them back where they belong.

Pros

+ *Taste*—The taste of natural, grass-fed beef can't be beat.

+ *Price*—The average cost of grass-fed beef in our area is around six dollars per pound, including the expensive cuts of steak. The hanging weight on our first grass-fed steer was just over three hundred pounds. At six dollars per pound this would value at $1,800, which far exceeds what we spent to raise him. It cost us $300 to purchase our steer, and it ate only pasture (plus supplemental hay in the winter). We ended up saving over $1,000 to raise our own grass-fed beef!

> **EVERYDAY NATURAL FARM TIP**
>
> To keep your beef cattle healthy, practice the following measures:
>
> • Provide a stress-free environment.
>
> • Monitor their feed consumption.
>
> • Keep an eye out for changes in vital signs.
>
> • Create a vaccination schedule and follow it.

+ *Peace of mind*—I love knowing exactly what our cows are being fed. We buy our hay from local fields that I know haven't been sprayed with pesticides. And we care for our cattle humanely.

Methods of raising cattle

We will discuss raising cattle and how to prepare your pasture at greater length in the next chapter. Here I want to explain the two primary methods you may want to use to raise your beef: organic or grass-fed.

There is some overlap between organic and grass-fed beef, as both methods are dedicated to raising healthier cows that are less chemically contaminated. However, not every pasture-raised cow is USDA certified organic, and not every organic cow is fed a 100 percent grass diet. If you are trying to decide between the two methods, make sure you understand what each label means and how each will impact the feed choices you make.[12]

Grass-fed

"Grass-fed" indicates that cattle are allowed to forage and graze for their own fresh food. They are likely to be given a substitute such as alfalfa during the winter, but the main focus is to provide as natural a diet as possible. Grains have more calories and cause the cows to grow faster at less cost, but grass has more key nutrients such as omega-3 fatty acids and B vitamins.[13]

Organic

The "organic" label tells you more about what cannot be used as feed to raise the cattle than it does about what to use. Your cows cannot be kept in a feed lot for any long period of time, and they cannot be overcrowded or kept in unsanitary conditions. They also cannot be exposed to antibiotics, hormones, GMOs, artificial pesticides, fertilizers, or other synthetic contaminants, whether directly or indirectly.[14]

Choosing either grass-fed or organic methods of raising beef will give you the same result—you'll be taking a big step toward improving your family's health and ensuring the welfare of the animals you raise. It is a big step to care for animals on a homestead, but it is very possible. In the next chapter we will further explore how to care for your animals, including going into more detail about how to make organic feed for them so they can provide the best quality meat, dairy, and eggs for your family.

Chapter 14

CARING FOR THE ANIMALS YOU RAISE

*I*N THE LAST chapter I introduced you to the possibility of raising some of your own poultry and farm animals. I included some easy ways to supply natural feed and offered tips for raising the kinds of animals common on natural farms.

In this chapter I want to take a closer look at just what is involved in the care and maintenance of farm animals. This will include all of the following:

+ More in-depth information on feeding animals naturally
+ A look at the different options for providing shelter for your animals
+ A look at the kind of attention animals must be given to keep them healthy

Let's get started.

FEEDING YOUR ANIMALS NATURALLY

Just as you are taking steps to feed your family healthy, natural foods, it is best to raise farm animals on organic, natural feed that is free from the chemicals and pesticides found in traditional animal feed. We will begin by reviewing some of the dangers of using traditional feed and then explore some natural, healthy options.

Traditional feed dangers

Today livestock raised for food are treated with drugs. The thinking is that these drugs are needed for the animals' health. However, the drugs used in animal populations have been associated with negative health effects in humans.[1]

There are five major classes of drugs given to food animals:

1. *Antiseptics, fungicides, and bactericides,* which treat skin or hoof infections, cuts, and abrasions when applied topically[2]

2. *Ionophores,* which alter rumen fermentation patterns, increase feed efficiency, and protect against some parasites[3]

3. *Steroid anabolic growth promoters,* which increase growth rate and the efficiency by which feed eaten is converted into meat, and peptide production enhancers such as recombinant bovine somatotropin (rBST) to increase milk production in dairy cows[4]

4. *Antiparasite drugs,* which are used to resist parasites[5]

5. *Antibiotics,* which are used to control diseases and promote growth[6]

These are the primary drug categories, but other drugs are used to prevent cattle from developing dangerous rumen-foam and bloat, to treat water to reduce the chances of infection in fish and shellfish, and to treat specific conditions.[7]

EVERYDAY NATURAL FARM TIP

Cattle can benefit from essential oils during the summer months, as oils protect them from heat stress and pesky insects. Flies, fleas, and lice irritate cattle. Strongly scented essential oils such as rosemary, cedar, lavender, and eucalyptus naturally repel pests and lessen the stress on the herd.

Providing organic feed for your poultry

Our free-range and pasture-raised chickens eat a lot of forage. They are constantly finding bugs and grasses, but they will peck at anything, including any garden vegetables I might be growing. So we keep them away from the areas where they just cannot forage. We give them a lot of table scraps, but we also supplement their diets with organic, natural feeds when necessary.

A benefit of raising your own chickens is that they give you organic eggs and meat. But as bloggers have noted, it can be nearly impossible to get organic chicken feed, and what is available is expensive. You can order it online or have it special-ordered by a feed store, but that approach is inconvenient. You will still likely pay less than you would for commercially raised poultry feed, but homesteaders are constantly looking for ways to save money.[8]

It is entirely possible to make your own organic poultry feed. I'm going to share one recipe found online, but you will want to do your own research to find more.

Homemade Poultry Feed Mix[9]

2 parts whole corn
3 parts soft white wheat
3 parts hard red winter wheat
½ part diatomaceous earth (not the kind you put in your pool)
1 part hulled barley
1 part oat groats
2 parts sunflower seeds
½ part peanuts
1 part wheat bran
1 part split peas
1 part lentils
1 part quinoa
1 part sesame seeds
½ part kelp

Mix the feed by hand so it is thoroughly incorporated. It doesn't hurt to run your hands through it before you give it to your poultry in case something settles.

When you make your own organic poultry feed, you can control everything that goes into it. Don't make huge amounts at one time so you can keep it fresh. Be sure to store your homemade feed in an airtight container.

EVERYDAY NATURAL FARM TIP

Comfrey, an herb we grow in our garden, traditionally has been used as livestock food. Dry comfrey contains protein and an assortment of healthy minerals. Because it is lower in fiber, it is a good feed for pigs and chickens that have trouble digesting fiber. It has also proven to be an excellent feed for horses, cows, donkeys, sheep, and goats.

Providing organic feed for your goats

I gave you some basic goat-feeding tips in the last chapter. Here we will look closer at the kinds of organic feed you want to supply to your goats.

Contrary to popular belief, goats do not eat everything in sight. They are, in fact, picky eaters. Their diet should consist mainly of hay. A goat's stomach is not designed to handle large amounts of grain, and too much can cause health problems. A small cupful in the morning and evening along with plenty of fresh dry hay will suffice. Hay dried in the sun in a location where there has been no rain is best. If there is rain, the hay may be wet inside and can mold. And be sure that the hay is kept in a manger. Most goats will not eat food that has fallen on the ground.

If you are raising dairy goats—goats from which you will be using and/or sharing raw goat's milk—keep in mind that organic livestock may be fed only ingredients that are certified organic. This means that the hay, grain, milk replacer, minerals, and supplements given cannot be genetically modified or contain antibiotics, synthetic hormones, or other restricted materials. You should not give any of those additives to your goats either.[10]

> Our free-range and pasture-raised chickens eat a lot of forage. They are constantly finding bugs and grasses, but they will peck at anything, including any garden vegetables I might be growing.

You may find a local feed mill that will partner with a nutritionist to create a custom feed mix using organic ingredients. If the feed mill is truly local, your shipping costs should be limited. Another option is to form a cooperative with others who are interested in obtaining custom organic goat feed. By doing so, you could have large quantities made at one time. It may take time to work out all the kinks, but forming a cooperative with like-minded farmers could be well worth the effort.[11]

If buying custom feed isn't your speed, you can find several homemade recipes for goat feed online. I am going to give you one option, and I recommend that you keep looking to find the one that best satisfies your own goats.

Homemade Dairy Goat Feed[12]

50 lb. of rolled barley
50 lb. of oats (whole, crushed, or rolled)
3 lb. of linseed meal
1 lb. kelp meal
Molasses to coat everything

This will make a lot of feed. You may want to use a big, clean tarp (a ten-by-twelve-foot tarp will work great) and a clean leaf rake to mix your grain. Dump the oats and barley onto the tarp and mix it all together with the rake. When your grain is thoroughly mixed, scatter the linseed meal and kelp meal over it and spread it out. If you overmix at this point, the linseed meal and kelp will sift to the bottom, which makes the next step a bit harder.

Now you will want to pour molasses over the grain and mix that in until your grain is well coated but slightly sticky. The amount of molasses you use will differ with each mixture. It usually takes about twelve cups to coat more than one hundred pounds of feed. Try starting with ten cups and work your way up from there.

Store your grain carefully! Large trash cans work well. If properly stored, the grain will keep for a month or more.

Providing feed for your cattle

If you want healthy, grass-fed beef, you'll need to pay attention to the health of your pasture, for this is what your cattle will be eating as long as the weather allows. If the climate where you live is good for keeping cattle on pasture, you may want to consider making your own hay for the winter months.

Hay is much less expensive for cattle than commercial grains. It is also digested more easily and contains more nutrients.[13] The quality of your hay will depend on the quality of your soil—how it is being cared for and what nutrients can be found within it. Here are a few general rules for growing hay:[14]

1. Instead of growing a single crop, grow a combination of legumes and grasses to ensure that you have a sufficient

supply. Legumes generally provide more protein, calcium, and magnesium than grasses do.

2. Though legumes are a useful crop to grow for hay, grass will help reduce the risk of bloat from legumes. It also helps speed the hay's drying process and keep the legumes upright, making them easier to cut.

3. Most cows prefer to eat mixed feeds as opposed to single crops. Keep in mind that both the land and cattle can benefit if the livestock are moved between different pastures (a practice called rotational grazing).

If you don't cut hay from your own pasture, buy cattle feed for the winter with utmost care. Make sure it has a good color and doesn't have any dampness, mold, or foul odors. Also check the core of the bale to ensure that the hay is crispy, pale green, and doesn't snap when bent.[15]

PROVIDING SHELTER FOR YOUR FARM ANIMALS

When we purchased our farm, we were blessed that it already had a wonderful barn to shelter our goats, a chicken coop, and ready homes for our pigs. But we had to build shelters for our other farmyard friends, including a duck house, turkey roost, pens for our meat rabbits, chicken incubators, buck area for our male breeding goats, and access to shelter for our sheep and cattle.

Making sure that all the animals we are raising on our Gather Heritage Farm have a place to live has been an interesting adventure. All farm animals need shelter for both summer and winter conditions. They need shade in the summer and protection from wind, rain, and severe cold.

There are hundreds of creative solutions for your animal shelters. I have heard of people building mobile chicken tractors from materials pulled from trash receptacles; chicken coops from discarded wood pallets; goat sheds from an old children's playhouse, old storage sheds, and recycled wood; and even elaborate shelters from expensive farm supplies. Whatever material the shelter is made of, its mission is to keep your animals stress-free and safe from predators and the elements.

The most common form of animal shelter is, of course, a barn. A barn serves three basic functions: to shelter livestock, store feed and equipment, and provide a place for you to repair your farm equipment. But for me, there is a fourth function—my barn just makes me feel good! If you are able to build a barn for your animals, be sure to combine your dream barn ideas with plenty of practical, realistic features that will save you money and prepare it for active use.[16]

When you are planning and budgeting for a new barn, keep in mind that you can add items later on. You don't have to include every element of your dream barn at the outset. However, some of the more modern conveniences you might want to consider for your barn include the following:[17]

+ Solar power
+ Hot water
+ Restroom
+ Overhead retractable hose with pressure nozzle
+ Rubber stall mats
+ Fly traps
+ Owl/bat houses
+ Cordless phone
+ Refrigerator
+ Space for a small tractor

We love our barn and recognize how fortunate we are to have one. We have thoroughly enjoyed building the additional shelters we needed for our farmyard menagerie, and we believe that we have the happiest farm animals in the mountains of North Carolina!

KEEPING YOUR ANIMALS HEALTHY

Livestock (and pet) owners are guardians of their animals and therefore have a moral obligation to give them the best care possible. Fortunately, as veterinarian Randy Kidd wrote, maintaining healthy livestock is neither an impossible nor an overly time-consuming task. He offers some "rules of the animal health road,"

> Keeping your animals healthy requires you to think ahead.

which he says "are guaranteed to help keep any cow, cur, goat, or guinea absolutely fit."[18]

He calls these "The Ten Commandments for Healthy Livestock." I will give you the abbreviated version of these commandments, but I encourage you to thoroughly research all aspects of your animal health concerns before you begin raising your animals.[19]

1. *Recognize your market*—Before you purchase farm animals, take a careful look at who will be eating their meat or using the milk, eggs, or whatever they produce.

2. *Know what a normal animal looks and feels like*—After you decide what kind of livestock to raise, make sure you can readily recognize healthy specimens of those breeds.

3. *Buy the best animals*—If your goal is to receive top production from your livestock (and it should be), you must buy the best animals available.

4. *Cull the worst animals*—In addition to choosing the best animal specimens, you must also avoid bringing the worst into your pens and pastures.

5. *Be aware of your animals' cycles*—Every animal has natural life patterns that govern them. You should know what those are.

6. *Keep meaningful records.*

7. *Build your animal housing well*—Once you have chosen the best livestock, your next responsibility will be to care for them well. That includes making sure they have safe, reliable shelter.

8. *Feed the critters correctly*—Animals need protein, carbohydrates, fat, vitamins, minerals, and water just as we humans do. You should know the specific requirements each animal needs to have a balanced diet.

9. *Coddle the "youngsters"*—Keeping your baby animals healthy is the most important thing you can do to remain in the livestock business for years to come. So spoil those cute little creatures.

10. *Help your animals prevent their own disease*—Each bird and beast must be protected against their species-specific diseases. The following tips will help you do just that:

+ Be sure that your animals' environment is carefully cleaned. Kidd notes that "if cleanliness is next to godliness, dirtiness is next to disease."[20]

+ Be careful not to bring illness onto your farm. Ensure that the animals you buy are not sick, and quarantine newcomers for a few weeks when you bring them onto your homestead to ensure that they aren't carrying some undetected disease. Also, wear boots when you visit the livestock areas on other farms and disinfect that footwear when you leave.

+ Keep in mind that parasites and local bugs are your animals' biggest enemies, so set up a good system with your local veterinarian to control worms and get your animals vaccinated as needed.

As you can see, these commandments for raising healthy livestock don't involve a lot of grueling extra work. You can keep your animals healthy with minimal fuss (which works for me because I am a minimalist!). However, keeping your animals healthy does require you to think ahead.

You've likely heard the saying, "An ounce of prevention is worth a pound of cure." Kidd rewrites it this way: "When it comes to keeping livestock well and productive, an ounce of prevention comes from using that pound of gray matter between your ears!"[21]

If you keep your animals healthy, they will be able to do their job well and nourish you and your family to the best of their ability.

Part V

Everyday Natural Family

Chapter 15

RAISING NATURAL, WHOLESOME, HOPE-FILLED CHILDREN

S OME DAYS I sit on my front porch wearing my comfortable "jammies" (my favorite old T-shirt and yoga pants), with my hands wrapped around a hot cup of bulletproof coffee and an old handmade afghan thrown over my shoulders, and watch my two children playing on their tire swing or running wild in the nearest pasture. In those moments I am overwhelmed with joy that I am able to raise everyday natural children in this world which has robbed so many parents of that joy.

I have to remind myself that raising everyday natural children is not something that comes naturally to parents today. Every aspect of raising everyday natural children has to be carefully thought out, planned, and orchestrated daily, or that dangerous outside world can easily infiltrate and rob us of the opportunity to keep our kids filled with health, happiness, and hope.

Of all the things about which I am most passionate, raising an everyday natural family is right at the top of the list. I'm pretty sure that is also true for you if you are reading this book. So in this chapter I want to share some tips for doing just that.

Two of my happiest days were the days our daughter and son were born. They were also two of the scariest days! There weren't any "how to raise everyday natural children" courses I could take or any cool and informative "mothering for dummies" classes available to prepare me to raise these two beautiful blessings from God.

But I think most of us forget that our Creator has prepared us, even if we do not feel prepared. Look at what He already did for every one of us:

You made all the delicate, inner parts of my body and knit them together in my mother's womb. Thank you for making me so wonderfully complex! It is amazing to think about. Your workmanship is marvelous—and how well I know it. You were there while I was being formed in utter seclusion! You saw me before I was born and scheduled each day of my life before I began to breathe. Every day was recorded in your book!

—Psalm 139:13–16

He started at the beginning with me. Before I even emerged into this world, He completely formed me, scheduled every day of my life, and recorded those days before they even happened. So as I sat as a new mother holding my first child, scared to bits about the task of doing a good job raising her, He had already scheduled every day and everything I would do on each of those days to raise her. I know, it's a lofty thought. But it helps me to rest a little bit and trust my intuition (another word for my God-given preparation for motherhood) about how to keep these two wonderful blessings natural and wholesome in today's frenetically unnatural and unwholesome world.

So let's start at the beginning and look at some of the *beginning* steps we can take to raise everyday natural children.

A Natural Cloth Diaper System

One thing I wanted to do with my babies was to use cloth diapers* instead of disposable ones, which are made with a list of dangerous ingredients. Research has proven that there are several potentially harmful chemicals in some disposable diapers, such as chlorine, fragrances, phthalates (chemicals used to soften plastic), dyes, and more.[1] Since the mid-1980s disposable diapers have included super absorbent polymer (SAP), which is referred to by an array of names including hydrogel, sodium polyacrylate, polyacrylate absorbents, and absorbent gel material.[2] It's not really clear whether sufficient testing has been done on SAP to ensure that it is nontoxic and safe. Most of the SAP being used today comes from petroleum, meaning it may have concerning chemical components.[3]

After doing a lot of research that convinced me there were safety issues with disposable diapers, and after doing the math to discover how much more money it would cost to use disposables, I ordered my first cloth diapers and gave them a try on my daughter.

I fell in love! She looked so cute, and they were so easy to use. (My favorite are the bumGenius diapers.* I never had any issues with them and used them through the diaper stages with both my children.) Over the next few weeks I developed a cloth diaper system that worked for me. I no longer need to diaper my kids, but I would recommend that you consider this option for your own everyday natural seedlings.

For my cloth diaper system, I kept a basket of cloth wipes* on the changing table, which we were able to keep near the sink. It was easy to wet them with warm water when I needed to use them. After I used them, I just threw them into the large diaper "wet bag" next to the changing table. All my cloth diapers were stored underneath the changing table for easy access. All the wet diapers went into the wet bag along with the cloth wipes.

So what about the poop? I used a diaper sprayer, which I highly recommend. It attaches to the toilet, and you just spray the poop off. I had a "nappy bucket" next to the toilet that locked, and that's where I tossed the poopy diapers. At nighttime I added thick inserts in the diapers to keep my little ones dry through the night.

I also developed a very easy system for washing the cloth diapers:

1. I threw all the diapers from the poop bucket and the large wet bag into the washer.

2. I washed them on the longest cycle, in warm water, without soap.

3. When the cycle was over, I washed them again in *hot* water, this time adding soap. (I now use Ecos detergent and have no problems.)

4. When the second cycle is over, I run the diapers through another rinse cycle. This gets rid of any detergent left on the diaper.

That's it! I hope you will give this cloth diaper system a try for your own natural everyday little ones. I love converting people to the cloth diapering method!

Feeding Your Baby Naturally

I provided breast milk for my babies and never had to give them any conventional baby formula. I firmly believe breast milk is the only milk a baby should get.

I was not challenged in that belief with my daughter, and though I had some serious difficulties nursing her, I was able to provide her with the breast milk I knew she needed. It was a different story with my son.

The day my sister died, my milk supply immediately tanked. I could no longer give my son the life-enriching breast milk he so needed. I was almost hopeless, ready to sacrifice the best for that conventional formula. In fact, there were a few days or weeks when I had to do just that. But then I received my miracle.

We think miracles are flying angels or supernatural healings or someone walking out of a wheelchair. But I've come to realize they aren't always like that. Miracles come in the form of plastic baggies, Styrofoam coolers, and little notes saying, "Ten ounces is all I could pump." They come in the form of a stranger handing you a cooler of pumped breast milk and giving you a hug. They come in the form of friends pumping while nursing their babies and then giving you their milk. They come in the form a UPS man handing you what looks like a regular package, but you know that inside there is two months' worth of breast milk for your baby that you weren't able to produce.

I have a new appreciation for the community of nursing mothers who donate their milk. They pump, and they nurse their own babies, and they drive fifty miles to give you something you so desperately need. They don't ask questions and don't ask for anything in return. And when you give them flowers to say thank you, they say they didn't think twice about it. My son is thriving today because of those mothers.

If you would like to be one of the mothers who can donate some of your precious breast milk to those who desperately need it, please contact the Human Milk Banking Association of North America (www.hmbana.org) to locate the milk bank closest to you.

As my children grew, I embraced the concept of baby-led weaning, which means letting your baby feed herself. You put out the food for them to grab, and they feed themselves. This approach does away with pureed foods. In essence you give chunks of food for the baby to gnaw on. No spoon is involved. No ice cube trays. No time spent making homemade pureed baby food. No money spent on expensive homemade baby food equipment. You give your baby what you are eating in pieces that she is able to pick up and eat.

> When my son started grabbing at my plate and sticking my food in his mouth, I knew he was ready to get some food of his own.

When my son started grabbing at my plate and sticking my food in his mouth, I knew he was ready to get some food of his own. I already knew I wanted to practice baby-led weaning with him, and for me at that time of our family life, it meant finding a way to do it the Paleo way.

One of the negatives about spoon-feeding babies is that they do not control how much food is put into their bellies. Often they have issues with constipation, gas, and the feeling of being overfull. With baby-led weaning, the baby is allowed to suck and lick his food in large chunks. He controls what he swallows. She is able to learn from the beginning how to properly chew her food. When they are spoon-fed pureed food, babies don't learn how to chew their food from the start. You have to teach it to them much later in their toddlerhood, which can be very frustrating.

I chose baby-led weaning for several reasons:

1. I was attracted to this concept because we were eating whole foods—no canned or frozen dinners. I knew I didn't want to give my son cereal as a first food because of all the information I had read on how terrible cereal was as a first food for a baby. Not only does it replace healthier foods, but babies can't digest grains well.[4] Plus, I wasn't eating grains because of their negative effect on my body, so why would I give my child grains as a first food?

2. It is a lazy (easy) way to feed your child! Seriously, baby-led weaning was so easy. The concept is to give your child what you are eating. And the best thing about this is that it forces you to eat healthily because your baby is going to be eating the same food!

3. Going out to a restaurant became so simple. And with a two-year-old and an infant in tow, I needed easy. I didn't have to pack a small cooler with pureed foods for my son. I fed him off my plate!

4. Baby-led weaning saved me time. Instead of spending hours pureeing his food, freezing it, and then thawing it to serve, I spent that time making a healthy meal for the whole family. There were times when I would mash the food up for him, but he never let me spoon-feed him.

5. Two of the top allergies among infants and toddlers are—drum roll, please—dairy and gluten. Eggs are also pretty high.[5] So I wanted to avoid these altogether.

I found that my son was naturally drawn to the taste of real food. I recommend that you try this way of weaning your child to real food. Introduce solid foods slowly and watch for any allergies. Wait at least four days after you've given your baby a new food before introducing another. Here are some of the foods that Sally Fallon, author of *Nourishing Traditions: The Cookbook That Challenges Politically Correct Nutrition and Diet Dictocrats*, recommends you begin with the following:[6]

+ Pastured egg yolk and bone stock
+ Avocado
+ Sweet potato
+ Squash of all kinds
+ Carrots
+ Broccoli and cauliflower (but be careful of gas)
+ All other vegetables
+ Meats of all kinds (we started with roasted chicken legs)
+ Banana, papaya, and pears
+ Other fruits

As parents there are a few things in life that we just can't control much, and one of them is what your children choose to eat. You can force-feed, which I don't recommend, but mealtimes will be more fun if you just let your baby guide you in what he or she will eat. By starting them early on healthy foods, you will give them a love for real, whole foods.

HOUSEHOLD CHORES FOR KIDS UNDER SEVEN

Raising everyday natural children means a lot of things, but it doesn't mean raising a kid to be a TV and video game–addicted couch potato. Unfortunately that's exactly what can happen unless we learn how to motivate our kids to better pursuits. One of the best ways to inspire kids to do more than sit in front of the tube is to teach them how to become creative, productive contributors to the household. Kids want to feel like they are part of what you're doing.[7] Getting them to start doing household chores may take some prodding, but you'll find that it's worth it in the long run.

> By starting them early on healthy foods, you will give them a love for real, whole foods.

My eight-year-old has been helping me with my essential oil tasks since I began. She has also already become Little Miss Farmer and gathers eggs, picks flowers, finds new vegetables growing on our farm, takes care of the chickens, gets sunflower seeds ready for roasting, and helps me cook and bake. She has even learned to crochet using the wonderful wool we harvested from our own Jacob sheep. My son loves to search for our free-range chicken eggs, help pick

EVERYDAY NATURAL TREATS FOR KIDS

You can easily make homemade popsicles for the kiddos with just a few ingredients, a blender, and some time. Just combine the ingredients using a blender until smooth, pour into popsicle molds, and freeze for three to four hours or until set.

FUDGESICLES

1 cup full-fat coconut milk

2–3 Tbsp. cocoa powder

1 large or 2 small bananas

1 tsp. vanilla

STRAWBERRY WATERMELON POPSICLES

¼ cup full-fat coconut milk

3 cups watermelon

1 cup strawberries

berries (yes, he eats most of them!), and help his father take care of the livestock.

Kids are not born with a work ethic. The character traits of tolerance, perseverance, and self-discipline are learned—and must be taught by us parents. It's up to us to teach our kids the difference between wanting and getting, and how to postpone gratification in order to accomplish and succeed later as an adult. In this section we will consider four aspects of planning and assigning chores to our little ones.

1. Motivate, but don't overwhelm your kids with chores.

Sometimes there is a fine line between motivating our children to do their chores and overwhelming them with demands and responsibilities, which will demotivate them. Here are a few dos and don'ts to keep in mind when giving your children chores:[8]

+ Don't insist on perfection.
+ Don't delay; begin assigning chores at an early stage.
+ Don't be stingy with praise.
+ Don't be inconsistent.
+ Do be specific with instructions.
+ Do ease into chores for children.
+ Do go easy with reminders and deadlines.
+ Do realize that your kids want to help.
+ Do remember that children have a short attention span.

2. Assign age-appropriate chores.

Our children are capable of doing so many more things than we even realize that it would be hard to give you an exhaustive list of everything your children can do at a specific age. You can do your own research to find many kinds of chores that might be appropriate for your children, but I would like to suggest several chores for each of three age groupings.

Chores for children aged two to three[9]

+ Putting toys away
+ Getting out and putting away a pet's food dish

+ Putting dirty clothes in the hamper
+ Wiping up their spills
+ Putting away their books and magazines

Chores for children aged four to five[10]
+ Brushing their hair and teeth
+ Making their own beds
+ Emptying wastebaskets
+ Pulling weeds if you have a garden
+ Clearing the table
+ Watering the flowers
+ Setting the table
+ Taking out the garbage

Chores for children aged six to seven[11]
+ Helping sort laundry
+ Sweeping the floors
+ Weeding
+ Raking leaves
+ Helping to make their school lunches
+ Keeping their bedrooms neat
+ Caring for pets
+ Helping to put away groceries

3. Consistently check up on your children's faithfulness.

Teaching kids about chores, money, and work is definitely a lifelong process. One of the most effective ways to inspire your children's faithfulness to their chores may be through the use of a chore chart. This can be used not only to provide motivation but also to help teach your children financial responsibility.

> Teaching kids about chores, money, and work is definitely a lifelong process.

Since children are much more excited about cute pictures than simple words, use a chore chart that is visually stimulating. You can do your own research and find many, many ideas for chore charts online.

You will want to place your chore chart in a visible location and make sure to review your children's accomplishments every day. Love, praise, and acknowledgment are your secret weapons to keep your children diligent to complete their chores.

4. Appropriately reward your children.

When you begin assigning chores to your children, be sure that you and your spouse have discussed what kinds of rewards or incentives you will be using. Maybe you think chores are just part of belonging to the family. As part of the family you expect them to chip in, help out, and do things around the house.

Even so, you may want to set up some kind of a reward system. It can be a powerful tool to motivate them. The rewards can be earned privileges, playdates, maybe a movie with a friend, or whatever you deem to be appropriate. Some parents will choose to reward their kids for their chores with money, thereby teaching important lessons about earning.

Since our children learn the most by watching us, be sure that you are modeling a positive work attitude yourself. Show pride in your accomplishments and share your insights with your kids. Let them see that your career is not just work; it's an opportunity to grow and achieve financial stability. Teaching your children to be independent and have life skills will allow them to feel empowered, and it will help them develop healthy self-esteem. Give your children every opportunity to be ready for whatever life brings them. That starts with simple household chores.

There is so much more involved with raising everyday natural children, but it will be different for each family. I hope this chapter gave you some ideas that will help you take your own first steps toward confidently raising everyday natural children. One thing I know is this: if even a few of us are successful at turning out kids who impact their world with ingenuity, confidence, integrity, and creativity, the world will become a better place to live. C'mon parents, we can do this together!

Chapter 16

NATURAL SOLUTIONS FOR CREATING ABUNDANCE

HERE WAS A point several years ago when my husband and I were faced with the financial problems that have become the normal way of life for many young couples. We had a pile of debt, including accumulated student loan debt, car payments, and rent payments, and for some reason we were contemplating getting wrapped up in more debt by taking on a mortgage.

Fortunately we found a way to get off the destructive path we were on. Someone in a Facebook group of mine was talking about financial coach Dave Ramsey. I had heard about him hundreds of time before, but this time something struck home.

My husband and I really wanted to get rid of some of our debt, so we sat down and wrote down each of our bills and the totals due, including our car and student loan debt. Thankfully we never had credit card debt, because the number was astounding.

Here we were, getting ready to purchase a house, and we had over $50,000 worth of debt to our name. And when I say about to purchase a house, I mean we had signed the offer and sent it to the seller's agent. The sellers made a counteroffer, and we had it in our hands about to sign when something told us to wait. We let the offer expire, and the whole deal fell through—thank the Lord! It turns out we didn't even want to live in the state where we were about to buy a house.

The jarring realization of how deep in debt we were prompted us to take a closer look at this whole Dave Ramsey thing. I kept hearing these Ramsey terms such as *snowball, baby steps,* and *emergency fund.* I spent the next few days researching his method and devising a plan to attack our debt. I hope this section gives you hope for getting out of debt, whether you make a ton of money or not.

When we began, we were $50,000 in debt. What was the catalyst for us to turn things around? I think it was when we actually sat down and wrote out each balance we had for each debt. We never thought of student loans as debt that should be paid off quickly. The same was true for car loans. However, we realized that debt is debt, and we wanted to get rid of it as soon as we could.

Most bank websites have a nifty tracking device that will let you categorize your spending. We noticed we were spending way too much on groceries (my fault) and eating out. Also, all the random things were adding up—and I couldn't even remember what most things listed on our statement were.

> Today we focus a little on cutting our spending and on boosting our income.

Using the Dave Ramsey materials as our guide, we sat down and made some critical decisions about the lifestyle adjustments we needed to make to get out of debt. Here are some of the steps we took.

+ We took the bank's tracking statement from our previous month and devised a plan to make each category significantly smaller.

+ We got rid of our iPhones (for more reasons than one) and signed up for prepaid phones through MetroPCS, which brought our $160 cell phone bill down to $60 per month. Part of our reason for getting rid of our iPhones is that we realized we were spending more time on them than with our kids. We decided that our family is more important. Did we miss them? Sure! However, we learned to hold each other's hands—"family hands," as my daughter calls them—instead of holding our phones.

+ We cut our cable and starting using Netflix and Hulu to stream shows on our Roku device. We bought an antenna to use if we wanted to watch broadcast television (newer TVs have this antenna built in).

- I joined a network marketing company and started selling essential oils to get as much money as I could on the side to help pay down debt.
- I stopped buying over-the-counter medication and cleaning products and started using essential oils instead.
- We called various customer service departments of several services we used (i.e., SiriusXM radio, car maintenance) and told them we couldn't afford the services anymore. They offered to reduce the payments by more than 75 percent!
- We made sure to reduce our electricity bill by turning off lights and not running the air conditioning too high.
- I make a lot of homemade cleaners to cut down on spending too much on store-bought products. (See chapter 11 for some ideas.)
- We bought (and still buy) almost everything used through Goodwill, Craigslist, and local thrift stores.
- We sold a *lot* of stuff. We sold a car, making us a one-car family. We sold furniture. We sold dishes, clothes, toys—anything we didn't really need.
- We started using the "envelope system" and took out cash for certain things such as my personal spending money, my husband's personal spending money, groceries, entertainment, and dining out. We used the cash for the week, and when it ran out, it was out.
- We stopped using our debit card and still only use it for gas.
- I strategically planned our meals by using a planning guide called Real Plans (realplans.com).

Thanks to Dave Ramsey's Financial Peace University, our family was able to pay off our debts and become financially stable. I highly recommend his materials, including his Financial Peace Junior resources, which are designed to help you teach your children how to win with money.

Today we focus a little on cutting our spending and on boosting our income. We have taken a journey through a direct sales essential oil company that has transformed our lives physically and financially. We felt such a difference using essential oils that I couldn't stop talking about them online and offline. So we partnered with this company and became distributors to help other people find natural solutions for their health, homes, and families.

I want others to experience the abundance and financial freedom my husband and I experience every day. We are living our dreams because we laid down a pipeline over the past four years and stopped hauling all those heavy and frustrating corporate buckets.

When I started with my essential oil company, we were heavy in debt but working toward becoming debt-free following the Dave Ramsey method. I was able to contribute a few thousand dollars a month to whatever debt we were working on getting rid of.

All the money from my blog and essential oil company went to paying down debt. We were adamant about getting the monkey of debt off our backs and determined to make it happen as soon as possible. We tore up bill after bill, and in April of 2014, we were debt-free! Two months later we called in to the Dave Ramsey radio show and screamed, "We are debt-free!"

Once we were debt-free and my entrepreneur income surpassed the income of my husband, we started talking about him coming home and working with me. We started dreaming again, and then we started living our dreams!

You see, our dream was to live in the mountains and have a farm. We wanted to raise our kids with wide-open spaces and live a life of freedom. We watched our dreams unfold right before our eyes and in June of 2015 were able to buy the farm of our dreams. My husband quit his busy corporate job, and now we work together on our business and are much happier!

STRATEGIC STEPS FOR STAYING OUT OF DEBT

You may not be led to follow the same path we followed to financial freedom. That is fine, because the purpose of this chapter is to help you realize that *staying out of debt* is just as important as getting out of debt. We believe everyone can do this, but it takes real effort, and not everyone will be able to use the same strategy. We have different lifestyles, different sources of income, different family needs, and different dreams and goals for our lives.

You are going to work hard in life, and if you have a dream, as we did, then you might as well work hard building your dream instead of your boss's. I want to leave you with eight strategic steps for staying out of debt that I believe will work for just about anyone.

1. Make an honest assessment of your spending and develop a budget that supports your family on the income you have available. A lot of people dread the idea of living on a budget that tells them when and how to spend every penny they make. But that's not really what a budget does. A budget is the fastest way to take control of your money, get out of debt, and begin moving toward your goals and dreams for your future.

   When we became debt-free and were ready to create a realistic budget for our debt-free life, we followed the principles in Dave Ramsey's book *The Total Money Makeover.* He has a great "Guide to Budgeting" tool available online that you can use to set up your budget.[1] There are others available, but this is the one that works best for us.

   > You are going to work hard in life, and if you have a dream, like we did, then you might as well work hard building your dream instead of your boss's.

2. Use the "envelope system" for your weekly cash needs. Every week we put the amount we have budgeted for weekly needs in envelopes—one envelope for each need. There is an envelope for my personal needs, my husband's personal needs, groceries, entertainment, and dining out. When the money runs out, it's out.

3. Carefully plan your grocery spending and meal planning for each week. As you know, we eat real, unprocessed food that is mostly organic. It is important to me to provide my family with whole foods that are nutritious, as natural as possible, and free of preservatives and other junk. This can be expensive, but I've developed some secrets to saving money while eating organic. Here are a few of them:

- I enrolled in an online meal planning service that sends me recipes each week and a grocery list![2]

- We raise our own meat chickens and egg-laying chickens. Before we raised chickens, I bought only whole chickens. I use every part—even the bones, which make delicious, healthy broth.

- Before we could raise our own beef cow, we bought our beef in bulk, purchasing one-fourth to one-half of a grass-fed cow at a time from a local farmer.

- I shop local and in season, using coupons wherever possible.

- We grow as many of our own fruits and veggies as possible and pick any produce we don't have in our garden.

- I save money in other areas of our life so I have money to splurge on healthy food.

4. Find economical ways to meet your family's wardrobe and home decorating desires. Frank and I are very frugal with our money, and we were both raised by parents who were penny-wise. My mother dragged my sister and me with her nearly every Saturday as she rounded the garage sale circuit. Most of our play clothes, toys, and home decorating items came from garage sales. No, they weren't old hand-me-downs. Many of them were originally high-priced items that had barely been used.

> **EVERYDAY NATURAL LIVING TIP**
>
> Even today, when it is much more possible for us to shop at first-rate stores, I buy much of what we purchase *used* from consignment shops, outlets, local thrift stores, and online websites.

5. Learn to make many of your personal-care products and home-cleaning products. I make as many products as possible. This is an important money-saving step that will free up money so you can reach your budget and savings goals.

6. Establish a regular method for putting money away into an emergency fund and savings plan. Frank and I are not

only concerned with having enough money to meet our needs today, but we are also determined to have a plan for emergencies big and small and savings for important things such as paying off our house, investing for our kids' college expenses, and preparing for our retirement.

We have learned that we will only save money when it becomes an emotional priority. It doesn't matter what you make—you can save money! We were motivated to start saving by studying Dave Ramsey's Financial Peace University. You can find one lesson on his website to whet your appetite for saving.[3]

7. Find an additional source of income that is home-based. Think about finding a creative way to bring more income into your life. When I first considered this, I began blogging. I wasn't sure how profitable it would be; I wanted to do it not only to earn income but also because I was passionate about the things I wanted to blog about. This is something you may want to try also.[4]

When I was introduced to essential oils, I became just as passionate about their value to my life and their potential for providing me with more income. Essential oils are volatile aromatic compounds extracted from plants, fruit, seeds, roots, and bark and have powerful health benefits. They can be used for a wide array of purposes for your health and home. It's important for you to know that it is their health-giving potential that fuels my passion to this day. They have indeed provided me with income far beyond what I anticipated, but that income only comes with determination, passion, and hard work![5]

8. Get rid of your credit cards. Credit card usage has become a way of life in America. Debt is the most aggressively marketed product in the history of the world.[6] Unlike Dave Ramsey, we are not suggesting that you get rid of every single credit card you have, but we are advising you to get rid of most of them and set boundaries on the one to three that you hang on to. That includes:

+ Only buying on credit when you have the cash to pay for the item

+ Paying off your credit card bill in full each month
+ Considering only using a credit card for recurring payments such as utility bills, cell phones, and other similar expenses

By doing that, you will not get imprisoned in credit card debt and the high interest rates that steal your money.

I want to close this chapter by sharing Dave Ramsey's seven characteristics of debt-free people.[7] Debt-free people are

+ wise,
+ patient,
+ confident,
+ goal-driven,
+ responsible,
+ not materialistic, and
+ willing to make sacrifices.

This describes who Frank and I want to be, and I hope you want to have these characteristics also. It is possible to truly enjoy your life without being a slave to debt. Being free to dream and create abundance is part of everyday natural living.

YOU CAN DO IT!

*N*ow that I've shared my journey to realizing my personal dreams—and much more than I ever could have dreamed—I want to ask you, are you dreaming? Have you opened up your mind and heart to recognize and visualize the person, the mother, the wife you want to be or the life you want your family to have? Or are you still afraid to really let yourself dream big?

My life changed the day I said yes to what I had only dared to imagine—an everyday natural life that allows us to eat wholesome foods, much of which we raise ourselves, and experience the freedom of being debt-free. Dreams remain just that until you put legs to them—until you take those first few baby steps onto the path that will lead you to make those dreams a reality.

Maybe your story is similar to mine. I didn't just need to take a first step into my dreams to be debt-free, live on a farm, and raise my children as simply and naturally as possible. I needed to take that first step out of the deep, deep hole of pain I was in because of the horrible, way-too-early death of my sister. Is there some kind of pain, sorrow, tragedy, or overwhelming, paralyzing crisis you can't seem to overcome?

Like turning a dream into a reality, turning pain and tragedy into joy and wholeness takes a first step. Mine came when I decided to lean on God's strength and gather up the scattered pieces of my life and then create the life I wanted.

That first step—and prayer—was all it took. The action of taking that first faltering step proved to be so much more powerful than the paralyzing, debilitating fear that had kept me from stepping out of my pain up to that time. From that first step I took many more steps, which included

+ making healthy dietary choices;
+ focusing on my health;

+ partnering with my husband to get out of debt;

+ bringing my husband home from his corporate job;

+ sharing my passion for essential oils with the world;

+ helping others take their first steps into realizing their dreams; and

+ giving back to our team and to charities we believe in.

I ask myself this question every day: "Why me, God? What did I ever do to deserve this sort of happiness?" And you know what? I realized I didn't have to do anything to deserve it. All I had to do was say yes! This life of hope, joy, and good health was His dream for me.

> "I long to accomplish a great and noble task, but it is my chief duty to accomplish small tasks as if they were great and noble."[1] —Helen Keller

Are you ready to say yes to your dreams? Stop sitting in the "no go" zone that can never lead you to realize your dreams. Stop being paralyzed by debilitating fears. Because *you can do it*!

To say yes to that dream, all you have to do is take your first faltering step. And then just determine that you will never stop. Take the second step, then the third step. Before you know it, you will find yourself walking right into the life you'd only imagined. Believe me. Believe the thousands of others who have taken that first step. Believe in yourself. You can do it!

RECOMMENDED RESOURCES

BEANS AND LENTILS

Azure Standard
www.azurestandard.com
Food-delivery service specializing in high-quality organic and natural products, including bulk beans and lentils

Adobe Milling
www.anasazibeans.com
Provider of heirloom beans and lentils

BUTTER AND GHEE

Kerrygold USA
www.kerrygoldusa.com
Provider of butter that comes from grass-fed cows in Ireland

Ancient Organics
www.ancientorganics.com
Provider of ghee from organic, grass-fed cows

Pure Indian Foods
www.pureindianfoods.com
Source of spiced ghee that is from organic, grass-fed cows

COCONUT PRODUCTS

Tropical Traditions
www.tropicaltraditions.com
Provider of coconut oil, coconut butter, and coconut flour

FATS AND OILS

Radiant Life (for Bariani Olive Oil)
www.radiantlifecatalog.com
Source of organic, first-pressed olive oil

Green Pasture
www.greenpasture.org
Provider of fermented cod liver oil, skate oil, and high-vitamin butter oil

FERMENTED FOOD STARTERS AND CULTURES

Cultures for Health
www.culturesforhealth.com
Provider of food cultures and starters for making yogurt, kefir, cheese, sourdough, and other fermented foods

FLOURS AND GRAINS

Jovial Foods
www.jovialfoods.com
Source for einkorn wheat berries and flour from nature's original wheat

Azure Standard
www.azurestandard.com
Food-delivery service co-op specializing in organic products and high-quality wheat, including einkorn, red wheat, and white wheat

FRUITS AND VEGETABLES

Local Harvest
www.localharvest.org
Offers connections to local farmers and CSAs (community supported agriculture programs) in your area

Pick-Your-Own
www.pickyourown.org
Offers connections to local farms where you can pick your own fruits and vegetables

GRASS-FED AND PASTURE-RAISED MEATS AND WILD-CAUGHT SEAFOOD

US Wellness Meats
www.grasslandbeef.com
Source of grass-fed beef and pasture-raised pork and chicken

Eat Wild
www.eatwild.com
Listing of producers of ethically raised meat in your area

The Brothery Bone Broth
www.bonebroth.com
Provider of bone broth from organic chickens or grass-fed cows

Vital Proteins Collagen and Gelatin
www.vitalproteins.com
Provider of sustainably sourced collagen and gelatin from grass-fed cows

GRASS-FED MILK

Campaign for Real Milk
www.realmilk.com
Listings of raw, grass-fed dairies around the United States

HOME AND KITCHEN SUPPLIES

Chicken Brooder
Brinsea EcoGlow Brooder (www.brinsea.com)

Digital Kitchen Scale
Ozeri Pronto Digital Multifunction Kitchen and Food Scale

Immersion Blender
Cuisinart Smart Stick CSB-75BC 200 Watt 2 Speed Hand Blender

Silicone Molds
Fat Daddio's Silicone Bakeware

Smart Pots
Smart Pots 50-Gallon Soft-Sided Container

Thermometers
Taylor Precision Products Classic Line Candy/Deep Fry Thermometer

NATURAL SWEETENERS

Organic Maple Syrup
Coombs Family Farms

www.coombsfamilyfarms.com
Provider of organic maple syrup and maple sugar products

Organic Sucanat
Wholesome Sweet
www.wholesomesweet.com
Provider of whole, unrefined cane sugar

Raw Honey
Bee Raw Honey
www.beeraw.com
Provider of raw honey that is unprocessed, unheated, and unfiltered

PERSONAL CARE

Ancient Minerals Magnesium Oil and Flakes
www.ancient-minerals.com
A revolutionary approach to magnesium supplementation

Cacao Butter, Shea Butter, and Beeswax
Mountain Rose Herbs
www.mountainroseherbs.com
A one-stop-shop for natural ingredients used to make homemade beauty products

Cloth Diapers
Cotton Babies
www.cottonbabies.com
A one-stop shop for all your cloth diapering needs, including bumGenius cloth diapers

Essential Oils and Diffusers
The Paleo Mama
http://thepaleomama.com/essential-oils/
Distributor of 100 percent pure, therapeutic-grade essential oils

Hair Care Products
Morocco Method
www.moroccomethod.com
Provider of a wide range of raw, wild-crafted hair-care products, including shampoo and conditioner, as well as henna, a safe and nontoxic way to dye your hair

SPICES AND DRIED HERBS

Mountain Rose Herbs
www.mountainroseherbs.com
Provider of organic spices, teas, and dried herbs

Redmond Real Salt
www.realsalt.com
Source of unrefined, natural sea salt

SUSTAINABLY CAUGHT FISH

Vital Choice
www.vitalchoice.com
Wild-caught salmon, shrimp, and other sustainable seafood options

BOOKS AND OTHER RESOURCES

Container Gardening
Edward C. Smith, *The Vegetable Gardener's Container Bible* (North Adams, MA: Storey Publishing, 2011).

Financial Freedom
Dave Ramsey, *The Total Money Makeover* (Nashville: Thomas Nelson, 2009).
Dave Ramsey, *Dave Ramsey's Financial Peace University* (New York: Vaughan Printing, 2004).
Dave Ramsey's Financial Peace Junior materials—www.daveramsey.com/store/.

NOTES

CHAPTER 2—LIVING AN EVERYDAY NATURAL LIFE

1. "Organic Foods: Are They Safer? More Nutritious?" Mayo Clinic, April 18, 2017, accessed May 11, 2017, http://www.mayoclinic.org /healthy-lifestyle/nutrition-and-healthy-eating/in-depth/organic-food/art -20043880?pg=1.

2. Jeffrey Skopek, "Thirty Pound Turkeys, Thirty Million Pounds of Antibiotics," *Harvard Law Bill of Health Blog*, November 27, 2013, https:// blogs.harvard.edu/billofhealth/2013/11/27/30-pound-turkeys-30-million -pounds-of-antibiotics/; Ethan A. Huff, "FDA: Thirty Million Pounds of Antibiotics Given to Conventional Livestock Annually," NaturalNews, October 9, 2013, accessed May 11, 2017, http://www.naturalnews .com/042401_FDA_antibiotics_conventional_livestock.html#.

3. "Where Can You Find Sustainable Food?," Grace Communications Foundation, accessed May 11, 2017, http://www.sustainabletable.org/566 /where-can-you-find-sustainable-food.

4. "Coop Directory Service Listing," accessed May 15, 2017, www .coopdirectory.org/directory.htm.

5. "Hydroponic Gardening for Beginners," Greentrees Hydroponics, accessed May 11, 2017, https://www.hydroponics.net/learn/hydroponic _gardening_for_beginners.asp.

6. "How to Build a Hydroponic Garden," WikiHow, accessed May 11, 2017, http://www.wikihow.com/Build-a-Hydroponic-Garden.

CHAPTER 3—EATING REAL FOOD

1. Courtney Dunkin, "What Is Real Food?," *Keeper of the Home* (blog), accessed May 12, 2017, http://www.keeperofthehome.org/what-is-real -food.

2. "Food Labels," Healthy Eating Advisor, accessed May 12, 2017, http://www.healthyeatingadvisor.com/food-labels.html.

3. Adrienne Santos-Longhurst, "The Health Benefits of Eating Real Food," *Little Green Pouch* (blog), February 27, 2014, https://www.littlegreen pouch.com/blogs/blog/12547697-the-health-benefits-of-eating-real-food.

CHAPTER 4—GROW IT, RAISE IT, OR BUY IT?

1.   Edward Group, "Seven Tips for Starting Your Own Organic Garden," Global Healing Center, June 6, 2009, last modified April 4, 2017, accessed July 10, 2017, http://www.globalhealingcenter.com/natural-health/gardening-tips/.

2.   Mark Whisnant and Patricia Whisnant, "Grass Fed Beef Hoax," Rain Crow Ranch, accessed May 16, 2017, https://www.americangrassfedbeef.com/grass-fed-hoax.asp.

3.   PETA.org, "Chickens Used for Food," accessed May 16, 2017, http://www.peta.org/issues/animals-used-for-food/factory-farming/chickens/.

4.   Joseph Mercola, "The Best Fish for Your Health and the Earth," Mercola, June 1, 2015, accessed May 12, 2017, http://articles.mercola.com/sites/articles/archive/2015/06/01/best-seafood.aspx.

5.   Ibid.

6.   Ibid.

7.   For more information about choosing healthy options in your local grocery store, see Stephanie Langford's "Nutritional Foundations" series at Keeper of the Home, accessed May 16, 2017, http://www.keeperofthehome.org/nutritional-foundations-making-the-best-of-the-regular-grocery-store.

8.   "The 2017 Dirty Dozen: Strawberries, Spinach Top EWG's List of Pesticides in Produce," Environmental Working Group, accessed May 16, 2017, https://www.ewg.org/foodnews/press.php.

9.   Ibid.

CHAPTER 5—DEVELOPING YOUR NATURAL EATING PLAN

1.   Joseph Mercola, "The Healing Benefits of Bone Broth," Mercola, September 22, 2016, accessed May 13, 2017, http://www.merliannews.com/The_Healing_Benefits_of_Bone_Broth/.

2.   "The Health Benefits of Raw Milk," Raw Milk Facts.com, last updated June 21, 2012, accessed May 13, 2017, http://www.raw-milk-facts.com/raw_milk_health_benefits.html; Josh Axe, "Raw Milk Benefits Skin, Allergies and Immunity," Dr. Axe, accessed May 13, 2017, https://draxe.com/raw-milk-benefits/; see also Virginia L. Barraquio, "Which Milk Is Fresh?," *International Journal of Dairy Science and Processing* 201, no. 1 (2014): 1–6.

3.   Don Colbert, *The Seven Pillars of Health* (Lake Mary, FL: Siloam, 2007), 189.

4.   Josh Axe, "20 Apple Cider Vinegar Uses," Dr. Axe, accessed May 13, 2017, https://draxe.com/apple-cider-vinegar-uses/.

5.   OrganicAuthority.com, "How to Use Apple Cider Vinegar For Beautiful Hair and Skin," HuffingtonPost.com, July 20, 2016, accessed May 16, 2017, http://www.huffingtonpost.com/organic-authoritycom/apple-cider-vinegar-beauty_b_1924171.html

6.   Jenny Hills, "How to Use Apple Cider Vinegar for Treating Arthritis," Healthy and Natural World, accessed May 13, 2017, http://www.healthyandnaturalworld.com /how-to-use-apple-cider-vinegar-for-treating-arthritis/.

7.   Axe, "20 Apple Cider Vinegar Uses."

8.   Bianca London, "The Incredible Uses for Apple Cider Vinegar Including Enhancing Your Workout, Boosting Weight Loss—and Even Calming Your CATS Down," DailyMail.com, May 7, 2017, accessed May 16, 2017, http://www.dailymail.co.uk/femail/article-4473976/The-incredible -uses-apple-cider-vinegar.html#ixzz4hHDDR0LN

9.   Axe, "20 Apple Cider Vinegar Uses."

10.   Joseph Mercola, "Coconut Oil: This Cooking Oil Is a Powerful Virus-Destroyer and Antibiotic," Mercola, October 22, 2010, accessed May 13, 2017, http://articles.mercola.com/sites/articles/archive/2010/10/22 /coconut-oil-and-saturated-fats-can-make-you-healthy.aspx.

11.   "Sweet Potatoes," The George Mateljan Foundation, accessed May 13, 2017, http://whfoods.org/genpage.php?dbid=64&tname=foodspice; see also Jacqueline Ritz, "Sweet Potato Breakfast Cookies: Flourless, Paleo and Grain Free," Wholistic Fit Living with Dr. Daisy Sutherland, accessed May 13, 2017, https://wholisticfitliving.com/sweet-potato-breakfast-cookies -flourless-paleo-grain-free?.

12.   Susan Napolitano, "Paleo Pumpkin Breakfast Cookies," The Preppy Paleo, September 27, 2012, accessed May 13, 2017, http://www .preppypaleo.com/2012/09/paleo-pumpkin-breakfast-cookies.html.

CHAPTER 6—DEALING WITH ISSUES OF WEIGHT

1.   Josh Axe, "Nine Charts That Show Why America Is Fat, Sick and Tired," Dr. Axe, accessed May 13, 2017, http://draxe.com /charts-american-diet/.

2.   Ibid.

3.   Ibid.

4.   Steve Kamb, "A Beginner's Guide to Healthy Eating," *Nerd Fitness* (blog), accessed May 13, 2017, http://www.nerdfitness.com/blog/2011/11/10 /healthy-eating/.

5.   Information in this section is adapted from "Nutrition: How to Make Healthier Food Choices," FamilyDoctor.org, accessed May 13, 2017, http://familydoctor.org/familydoctor/en/prevention-wellness/food-nutrition /healthy-food-choices/nutrition-how-to-make-healthier-food-choices.html.

6.   Tamar Haspel, "Is Grass-Fed Beef Really Better for You, the Animal, and the Planet?," *Washington Post*, February 23, 2015, accessed May 13, 2017, https://www.washingtonpost.com/lifestyle/food/is-grass-fed -beef-really-better-for-you-the-animal-and-the-planet/2015/02/23/92733524 -b6d1-11e4-9423-f3d0a1ec335c_story.html?utm_term=.f0de669a063b.

7.   Markham Heid, "Why Full-Fat Dairy May Be Healthier Than Low-Fat," *Time*, March 5, 2015, http://time.com/4279538/low-fat-milk -vs-whole-milk/; see also Markham Heid, "Why Full-Fat Dairy May Be Healthier Than Low-Fat," *Time*, March 5, 2015, http://time.com/3734033 /whole-milk-dairy-fat/.

8.   Adapted from "Weight Loss: Six Strategies for Success," Mayo Clinic, accessed May 14, 2017, http://www.mayoclinic.org/healthy-lifestyle /weight-loss/in-depth/weight-loss/art-20047752?pg=1.

9.   Gina DeMillo Wagner, "Build a Better Body Image," *Experience Life*, April 2012, accessed May 13, 2017, https://experiencelife.com/article /build-a-better-body-image/.

10.   "Ten Steps to Positive Body Image," National Eating Disorders Association, 2005, accessed May 14, 2017, www.NationalEatingDisorders .org, available at https://uhs.berkeley.edu/whatseatingyou/pdf/TenSteps BodyImage.pdf. Used with permission.

11.   Carmen Harra, "Thirty-Five Affirmations That Will Change Your Life," *The Huffington Post* (blog), September 5, 2013, http://www.huffington post.com/dr-carmen-harra/affirmations_b_3527028.html.

CHAPTER 7—EMBRACING NATURAL HYGIENE

1.   Einav Keet, "Cosmetics: The Good, the Bad, and the Ugly," Share Guide, accessed May 14, 2017, http://www.shareguide.com/cosmetics.html.

2.   Ibid.

3.   "Artificial Colors and Fragrance Woes," Bubble and Bee Organic, accessed May 14, 2017, http://bubbleandbee.com/artificial-colors-and -fragrance-woes/; see also Ruth Winter, *A Consumer's Dictionary of Cosmetic Ingredients*, 7th ed. (New York: Three Rivers, 2009), 402.

4.   Pat Thomas, "Behind the Label: Listerine Teeth and Gum Defence," Ecologist, January 13, 2009, accessed May 14, 2017, http://www .theecologist.org/green_green_living/behind_the_label/269558/behind_the _label_listerine_teeth_and_gum_defence.html.

5.   Edward Group, "Why You Should Use Aluminum-Free Deodorant," Global Healing Center, May 22, 2015, last updated June 8, 2015, http://www.globalhealingcenter.com/natural-health/why-you-should -use-aluminum-free-deodorant/.

6.   "Nature's Alternatives to Synthetics," OrganicGlow, accessed May 14, 2017, http://organicglow.com/about/educating-consumers/natures -effective-alternatives-to-synthetics/.

7.   Katherine Martinko, "Twenty Toxic Ingredients to Avoid When Buying Body Care Products and Cosmetics," *TreeHugger* (blog), February 25, 2014, accessed May 14, 2017, https://www.treehugger.com/organic- beauty/20-toxic-ingredients-avoid-when-buying-body-care-products-and -cosmetics.html; see also Gillian Deacon, *There's Lead in Your Lipstick:*

Toxins in Our Everyday Body Care and How to Avoid Them (Toronto, Ontario: Penguin Canada, 2010).

8. Ibid.

9. Stephanie Petersen, "Top Five Benefits of Using Natural Health and Beauty Products," Overstock, accessed May 14, 2017, http://www.overstock .com/guides/top-5-benefits-of-using-natural-health-and-beauty-products.

10. Ramiel Nagel, *Cure Tooth Decay* (Ashland, OR: Golden Child Publishing, 2010).

11. Weston A. Price, *Nutrition and Physical Degeneration*, 8th ed. (Lemon Grove, CA: Price Pottenger Nutrition, 2009).

12. Bruce Fife, *Oil Pulling Therapy* (Colorado Springs, CO: Piccadilly Books, 2008).

13. Annmarie Gianni, "What's the Difference Between Extra Virgin and Fractionated Coconut Oil?," Annmarie Skin Care, accessed May 14, 2017, https://www.annmariegianni.com/whats-the-difference-extra-virgin -and-fractionated-coconut-oil/; see also Nazimah Hamid, "Antioxidant Capacity of Phenolic Acids of Virgin Coconut Oil," *International Journal of Food Sciences and Nutrition* 60, Suppl. 2 (January 2009): 114–123.

14. See Appendix: Recommended Resources.

15. Jackie Ritz, "How to Order dōTERRA Essential Oils," *The Paleo Mama* (blog), accessed May 14, 2017, http://thepaleomama.com/essential-oils/.

CHAPTER 8—RADIANT SKIN

1. Ashley Welch, "Ten Amazing Facts about Your Skin," Everyday Health, last updated June 25, 2015, accessed May 14, 2017, http://www .everydayhealth.com/news/10-amazing-facts-about-skin/.

2. Ibid.

3. Ruta Ganceviciene et al., "Skin Anti-Aging," *Dermato-endocrinology* 4, no. 3 (2012): 308–319, doi:10.4161/derm.22804.

4. "Organic Spirulina 100 Percent Pure 1 Lb," National Nutrition, accessed May 14, 2017, http://www.nationalnutrition.ca/detail.aspx?ID=4567.

5. "The Eight Best Natural Ingredients for Your Skin," Everyday Health, last updated November 12, 2013, accessed May 14, 2017, http:// www.everydayhealth.com/beauty-pictures/the-8-best-natural-ingredients -for-your-skin.aspx#03.

6. Tiffany Ayuda, "Which Teas You Should Drink to Improve Your Skin," *Women's Health*, June 24, 2015, http://www.womenshealthmag.com /beauty/teas-for-better-skin; see also Steven D. Ehrlich, "Green Tea: Overview," University of Maryland Medical Center, November 6, 2015, http:// www.umm.edu/health/medical/altmed/herb/green-tea.

7.   Katie Wells, "Matcha Green Tea Face Mask Recipe," *Wellness Mama* (blog), February 28, 2017, http://wellnessmama.com/60288/green-tea-face-mask/.

8.   Crunchy Betty, "Nitty Gritty on the Oil Cleansing Method," *Crunchy Betty* (blog), last updated May 7, 2017, https://crunchybetty.com/oil-cleansing-method/.

9.   Ibid.

10.   Denorex Staff, "The History of Shampoo," *Denorex Dandruff and Scalp Care* (blog), March 24, 2015, http://www.denorex.com/blog/the-history-of-shampoo.

11.   June Kellum Fakkert, "Shampoo Ingredients You Want to Avoid," *The Epoch Times* April 12, 2014, last updated August 10, 2016, http://www.theepochtimes.com/n3/616834-shampoo-ingredients-you-want-to-avoid/.

12.   Kati Blake, "Shampoo Ingredients You Should Know About: 2. Formaldehyde," *All Women's Talk* (blog), accessed May 14, 2017, http://hair.allwomenstalk.com/shampoo-ingredients-you-should-know-about/2.

13.   Fakkert, "Shampoo Ingredients."

14.   Kati Blake, "Shampoo Ingredients You Should Know About: 3. Isopropyl Alcohol," *All Women's Talk* (blog), accessed May 14, 2017, http://hair.allwomenstalk.com/shampoo-ingredients-you-should-know-about/3.

15.   Fakkert, "Shampoo Ingredients."

16.   "Organic versus Non Organic Shampoo—What Are the Pros and Cons," *Talking Odours* (blog), May 5, 2012, https://h2odots.wordpress.com/2012/05/05/organic-versus-non-organic-shampoo-what-are-the-pros-and-cons/.

17.   Team TreeHugger, "Everything You Need to Know About Natural Skin Care," *TreeHugger* (blog), June 23, 2014, http://www.treehugger.com/htgg/how-to-go-green-natural-skin-care.html.

18.   "Stellar Organic Certification," Demeter Association, accessed May 14, 2017, http://www.demeter-usa.org/stellar-certification/.

19.   Jelena Jovanovic, "Nineteen Fantastic Natural Homemade Shampoos," *All Women's Talk* (blog), accessed May 14, 2017, http://hair.allwomenstalk.com/fantastic-natural-homemade-shampoos.

20.   Sadia, "Five Simple Conditioners for Damaged Hair," StyleCraze, June 26, 2016, http://www.stylecraze.com/articles/simple-homemade-conditioners-for-damages-hair/.

21.   "About Henna," Silk & Stone, accessed May 16, 2017, http://silknstone.com/About-Henna.html.

22.   "10 Unusual Uses of Henna and How to Use It on Hair," Positive Med, February 1, 2014, accessed May 16, 2017, http://positivemed.com/2014/02/01/10-unusual-uses-henna-use-hair/; see also Catherine Cartright-Jones, "Henna and Health," HennaforHair.com, accessed May 16, 2017, http://www.hennaforhair.com/health/.

23.   Jackie Ritz, "How to Dye Your Hair with Henna," *The Paleo Mama* (blog), November 11, 2013, accessed May 15, 2017, http://thepaleomama.com/2013/11/henna-hair-dye-safe-nontoxic/; see also Jackie Ritz, "Henna Hair Dye," *The Paleo Mama* (blog), April 1, 2012, accessed May 15, 2017, http://thepaleomama.com/2012/04/henna-hair-dye/.

CHAPTER 9—FINDING THE PATH TO NATURAL HEALTH

1.   Joseph Mercola, "Dr. Mercola's Natural Health Tips Infographic," Mercola, accessed May 14, 2017, http://www.mercola.com/infographics/natural-health-tips.htm.

2.   Ibid.

3.   "Find a Vitamin or Supplement: Elderberry," WebMD, accessed May 14, 2017, http://www.webmd.com/vitamins-supplements/ingredientmono-434-elderberry.aspx?activeingredientid=434&activeingredientname=elderberry; see also Josh Axe, "Elderberry: Natural Medicine for Colds, Flus, Allergies and More," Dr. Axe, accessed May 14, 2017, https://draxe.com/elderberry/.

4.   Ibid.

5.   "Using Elderberry as an Herbal Remedy," Every Green Herb, accessed May 16, 2017, http://www.everygreenherb.com/elderberry.html.

6.   A. L. Thomas et al., "'Marge': a European Elderberry for North American Producers," *Acta Hortic*, 2015: 191–199, viewed at https://www.ncbi.nlm.nih.gov/pmc/articles/PMC4863952/.

7.   MaryEllen, "Growing and Using Echinacea," Off the Grid News, 2012, accessed May 14, 2017, http://www.offthegridnews.com/alternative-health/growing-and-using-echinacea/; see also Lynn Hunt, "New Hybrid Coneflowers: How Reliable Are They?," *Christian Science Monitor*, July 12, 2011, http://www.csmonitor.com/The-Culture/Gardening/diggin-it/2011/0712/New-hybrid-coneflowers-How-reliable-are-they.

8.   Ibid.

9.   Ibid.; see also "Herbal Remedies for Sore Throat," The Herbal Resource, accessed May 14, 2017, https://www.herbal-supplement-resource.com/remedies-sore-throat.html.

10.   "Find a Vitamin or Supplement: Echinacea," WebMD, accessed May 14, 2017, http://www.webmd.com/vitamins-supplements/ingredientmono-981-echinacea.aspx?activeingredientid=981&.

11.   Anahad O'Connor, "The Doctor's Remedy: Turmeric for Joint Pain," *New York Times*, October 19, 2011, accessed May 14, 2017, http://well.blogs.nytimes.com/2011/10/19/the-doctors-remedy-turmeric-for-joint-pain/?_r=0.

12.   Krupa Vyas, "The Cure Is in the Roots: Turmeric," *Journal of Nutritional Disorders & Therapy*, https://www.omicsonline.org/open-access/the-cure-is-in-the-roots-turmeric-2161-0509-1000163.php?aid=52844.

13.   "Find a Vitamin or Supplement: Turmeric," WebMD, accessed May 14, 2017, http://www.webmd.com/vitamins-supplements/ingredientmono -662-turmeric.aspx?activeingredientid=662.

14.   Joseph Mercola, "Curcumin: The Spice That Is Better Than Drugs for Rheumatoid Arthritis," Mercola, June 13, 2012, accessed May 15, 2017, http://articles.mercola.com/sites/articles/archive/2012/06/13/the-spice-that -is-better-than-drugs-for-ra.aspx.

15.   Joseph Mercola, "What Is Golden Milk?," Mercola, September 21, 2015, accessed May 15, 2017, http://articles.mercola.com/sites/articles /archive/2015/09/21/golden-milk.aspx.

16.   Diana Kaniecki, "Turmeric for Back Pain," LiveStrong, October 14, 2015, http://www.livestrong.com/article/450412-turmeric-for-back-pain/.

17.   "Comfrey—The Homesteader's Gold Mine," Rise and Shine Rabbitry, August 11, 2013, accessed May 15, 2017, https://riseandshinerabbitry .com/tag/organic/?.

18.   "Three Big Reasons to Choose Natural Cures and Natural Remedies Over Orthodox Medical Treatments," Life-Saving Natural Cures and Natural Remedies, accessed May 14, 2017, http://www.life-saving-natural cures-and-naturalremedies.com/.

19.   John T. James, "A New, Evidence-Based Estimate of Patient Harms Associated With Hospital Care," *Journal of Patient Safety* 3, no. 9 (September 2013): 122–28, doi:10.1097/PTS.0b013e3182948a69, http:// journals.lww.com/journalpatientsafety/Fulltext/2013/09000/A_New,_Evi- dence_based_Estimate_of_Patient_Harms.2.aspx.

CHAPTER 10—HOMEMADE BODY-CARE WONDERS

1.   Josh Axe, "Goat Milk Benefits Are Superior to Cow Milk," Dr. Axe, accessed May 14, 2017, https://draxe.com/goat-milk/.

2.   Ibid.

3.   Jackie Ritz, "Traditional Goat Milk Soap Recipe," *The Paleo Mama* (blog), October 22, 2014, http://thepaleomama.com/2014/10/traditional -goat-milk-soap-recipe/.

4.   "How to Take a Detox Bath," WikiHow, accessed May 14, 2017, http://www.wikihow.com/Take-a-Detox-Bath.

5.   AJ Willingham, "What's the Tie between Talc and Cancer?" CNN, May 3, 2016, accessed May 15, 2017, http://www.cnn.com/2016/02/25/health /talc-safety-explainer-hln/.

CHAPTER 11—DETOXING YOUR HOME

1.   Alanna Ketler, "Top Eleven Spring Cleaning Products You Must Avoid," Natural Blaze, March 12, 2014, accessed May 14, 2017, http://www .naturalblaze.com/2014/03/top-11-spring-cleaning-products-you.html.

2. Ibid.; see also "Antibacterial Soaps: Being Too Clean Can Make People Sick, Study Suggests," Science Daily, November 30, 2010, accessed May 14, 2017, https://www.sciencedaily.com/releases/2010/11/10112910 1920.htm.

3. These tips were adapted from Alana Ketler, "Top Spring Cleaning Products and Chemicals to Avoid for Environmental and Health Reasons," Collective Evolution, March 12, 2014, accessed April 27, 2017, http://www .collective-evolution.com/2014/03/12/top-spring-cleaning-products-chemicals -to-avoid-for-environmental-health-reasons/.

4. This list was adapted from "Non-Toxic Home Cleaning," Eartheasy, accessed May 14, 2017, http://eartheasy.com/live_nontoxic_solutions.htm, and was edited for grammar and style.

5. "Borax," ToxNet, accessed May 14, 2017, https://toxnet.nlm.nih.gov /cgi-bin/sis/search/a?dbs+hsdb:@term+@DOCNO+328.

6. Marie Kondo, *The Life-Changing Magic of Tidying Up* (Berkeley, CA: Ten Speed Press, 2014).

7. Ibid.

8. "Non-Toxic Home Cleaning," Eartheasy.

9. Ibid.

10. "Natural Multi-Purpose Citrus Cleaner," *Lexie Naturals* (blog), October 20, 2011, accessed May 14, 2017, http://blog.lexienaturals.com /2011/10/natural-cleaning.html.

Chapter 12—Gardening Like the Master Gardener

1. "Vegetable Gardening: Ten Must-Grow Plants," Better Homes and Gardens, accessed May 14, 2017, http://www.bhg.com/gardening/vegetable /vegetables/10-must-grow-plants/.

2. "USDA Hardiness Zone Map," Better Homes and Gardens, accessed May 14, 2017, http://www.bhg.com/gardening/gardening-by-region /regional-gardening/hardiness-zone-map/.

3. "Garden Crops: Cold Storage Ideas and Root Cellar Tips," TipNut, accessed May 14, 2017, http://tipnut.com/cold-storage-projects/?.

4. "Successful Tips for Growing an Organic Vegetable Garden," Better Homes & Gardens, accessed May 16, 2017, http://www.bhg.com/gardening /vegetable/vegetables/tips-for-growing-an-organic-vegetable-garden/.

5. Lynn Bement, "Six Ways to Make Great Compost," *Fine Gardening* 130, accessed May 14, 2017, http://www.finegardening.com/6-ways -make-great-compost.

6. RidgeView, "Garden Harvest Tips," Ridgeview Garden Centre, August 20, 2015, accessed May 14, 2017, http://ridgeviewgardencentre.com /garden-harvest-tips/?.

7. Ibid.

8. Deborah Smith, "Yard2Kitchen Brings Organic Gardening Home," *Jersey Bites*, August 10, 2016, accessed May 14, 2017, https://jerseybites.com /2016/08/yard2kitchen-brings-organic-gardening-home/.

9. *Oxford Living Dictionaries*, s.v. "diatomaceous earth," accessed May 14, 2017, https://en.oxforddictionaries.com/definition/us/diatomaceous_earth.

10. "Spinosad: General Fact Sheet," National Pesticide Information Center, reviewed August 2014, accessed May 14, 2017, http://npic.orst.edu /factsheets/spinosadgen.html.

11. Barbara Pleasant, "Organic Pest Control: What Works, What Doesn't," June/July 2011, accessed May 14, 2017, http://www.motherearth news.com/organic-gardening/pest-control/organic-pest-control-zm0z11zsto.

12. "Nine All Natural Ways to Get Rid of Slugs in Your Garden," Plant Care Today, accessed May 15, 2017, https://plantcaretoday.com /naturally-get-rid-of-slugs.html.

13. Sarah, "Six Ways to Control Squash Bugs in Your Garden," *The Free Range Life* (blog), accessed May 14, 2017, http://thefreerangelife.com /control-squash-bugs/.

14. Jackie Carroll, "Killing Aphids Naturally: How to Get Rid of Aphids Safely," Gardening Know How, accessed May 14, 2017, http://www .gardeningknowhow.com/plant-problems/pests/insects/homemade-aphid -control.htm.

15. Amy Young Miller, "Six—Make that Seven!—Natural Ways to Get Rid of Nasssty Cabbage Moths!!," *vomitingchicken.com Blog*, December 6, 2014, http://vomitingchicken.com/natural-ways-to-get-rid-of-those-nasty -cabbage-moths/.

16. Marie Stegner, "Eco-Friendly Ways to Get Rid of Garden Pests," Your Organic Child, April 12, 2011, accessed May 14, 2017, http://your organicchild.com/eco-friendly-ways-to-get-rid-of-garden-pests/.

17. "Tips for Getting Rid of Tomato Hornworms," Veggie Gardener, July 5, 2009, accessed May 14, 2017, http://www.veggiegardener.com/tips -for-getting-rid-of-hornworms/.

18. Stegner, "Eco-Friendly Ways to Get Rid of Garden Pests."

19. Montana Homesteader, "How to Get Rid of Cutworms in the Garden," *Montana Homesteader Blog*, June 20, 2014, accessed May 14, 2017, http://montanahomesteader.com/get-rid-cutworms-garden/.

20. Gene Gerue, "Construct a Chicken Moat for Effective Garden Pest Control," Mother Earth News, May/June 1988, accessed May 14, 2017, http://www.motherearthnews.com/homesteading-and-livestock/garden-pest -control-zmaz88mjzgoe.aspx.

21. Heather Rhoades, "Controlling Cucumber Beetles—How to Deter Cucumber Beetles in the Garden," Gardening Know How, March 20, 2016, accessed May 14, 2017, http://www.gardeningknowhow.com/edible/vegetables /cucumber/cucumber-beetle-control.htm.

22. "Corn Earworm," Planet Natural Research Center, accessed May 14, 2017, http://www.planetnatural.com/pest-problem-solver/garden-pests/corn-earworm-control/.

23. "Whitefly," Planet Natural Research Center, accessed May 14, 2017, http://www.planetnatural.com/pest-problem-solver/houseplant-pests/whitefly-control/.

24. Richard P. King, "Save Vegetable Seeds in Your Backyard," September/October 1977, accessed May 14, 2017, http://www.motherearthnews.com/organic-gardening/save-vegetable-seeds-backyard-zmaz77zsch.

25. Mike and Nancy Bubel, "The Fundamentals of Root Cellaring," Mother Earth News, August/September 1991, accessed May 14, 2017, http://www.motherearthnews.com/real-food/root-cellaring/fundamentals-of-root-cellaring-zm0z91zsie.

26. Debbie Moors, "22 Foods You Can Store in Root Cellars," Hobby Farms.com, August 2, 2012, accessed May 16, 2017, http://www.hobbyfarms.com/22-foods-you-can-store-in-root-cellars-2/.

27. Bubel, "The Fundamentals of Root Cellaring," Mother Earth News,

28. Ibid.

CHAPTER 13—RAISING LIVESTOCK NATURALLY

1. Jody Padgham, "Introduction to Pastured Poultry," *Organic Producer*, July 1, 2014, accessed May 15, 2017, http://www.organicproducermag.com/index.cfm/fuseaction/feature.display/feature_id/358/index.cfm?.

2. Ibid.

3. Lauren Arcuri, "How to Process Chickens," The Spruce, April 12, 2017, accessed May 15, 2017, https://www.thespruce.com/slaughter-chickens-for-meat-3016856.

4. Carolyn Robinson, "Raising Geese for Meat and More," Mother Earth News, March/April 1970, accessed May 15, 2017, http://www.motherearthnews.com/homesteading-and-livestock/raising-geese-zmaz70mazglo.aspx.

5. Ibid.

6. "American Buff Goose," The Livestock Conservancy, accessed May 15, 2017, http://livestockconservancy.org/index.php/heritage/internal/buffgoose?.

7. Kris Wetherbee, "Raising Dairy Goats and the Benefits of Goat Milk," Mother Earth News, June/July 2002, accessed May 15, 2017, http://www.motherearthnews.com/homesteading-and-livestock/benefits-of-goat-milk-zmaz02jjzgoe.

8. Ibid.

9. Ibid.

10. Ibid.

11.   Melissa Norris, "Pros and Cons of Raising Your Own Grass Fed Beef," *Pioneering Today* (blog), March 20, 2013, accessed May 15, 2017, http://melissaknorris.com/raising-your-own-grass-fed-beef/.

12.   "Grass Fed Beef vs. Organic Beef," Topline Foods, accessed May 15, 2017, http://www.toplinefoods.com/grass-fed-beef-meat-vs-organic-beef-meat.

13.   Ibid.

14.   Ibid.

CHAPTER 14—CARING FOR THE ANIMALS YOU RAISE

1.   National Research Council, "The Use of Drugs in Food Animals: Benefits and Risks," The National Academy of Sciences (Washington DC: The National Academies Press, 1999). doi:10.17226/5137.

2.   Ibid.

3.   Ibid.; see also Matt Hersom and Todd Thrift, "Application of Ionophores in Cattle Diets," University of Florida Institute of Food and Agricultural Sciences, 2015, accessed May 15, 2017, http://edis.ifas.ufl.edu/an285.

4.   National Research Council, "Drugs in Food Animals"; see also "Steroid Hormone Implants Used for Growth in Food-Producing Animals," US Food and Drug Administration, last updated October 20, 2015, accessed May 15, 2017, https://www.fda.gov/AnimalVeterinary/Safety Health/ProductSafetyInformation/ucm055436.htm.

5.   National Research Council, "Drugs in Food Animals."

6.   Ibid.

7.   Ibid.

8.   Marye Audet, Planet Green, "Organic Chicken Feed Is Cheep When You Make It Yourself," How Stuff Works.com, January 11, 2012, accessed May 15, 2017, http://home.howstuffworks.com/green-living/organic -chicken-feed-cheap.htm.

9.   Ibid.

10.   Cheryl K. Smith, "How to Raise Dairy Goats for Organic Goat Milk," Countryside Daily, April 10, 2017, accessed May 15, 2017, http://countrysidenetwork.com/daily/livestock/goats/organic-goat-farming-basics -raising-organic-dairy-goats.

11.   Ibid.

12.   Goat Song, "How to Make Homemade Dairy Goat Feed," *To Sing With Goats* (blog), November 13, 2013, http://lifeatmennageriefarm. blogspot.com/2013/11/how-to-make-homemade-dairy-goat-feed.html.

13.   "Raising Grass Fed Beef Cattle," Raising Cattle for Beginners, March 17, 2013, accessed May 15, 2017, http://www.raising-cattle.com /raising-grass-fed-beef-cattle/?.

14.   Ibid.

15.   Ibid.

16.   Sarah Christie, "Build a Better Barn for Your Family," Hobby Farms, February 18, 2009, accessed May 15, 2017, http://www.hobbyfarms.com/build-a-better-barn-for-your-farm-3/.

17.   Ibid.

18.   Randy Kidd, "Ten Commandments for Raising Healthy Livestock," Mother Earth News, July/August 1979, accessed May 15, 2017, http://www.motherearthnews.com/homesteading-and-livestock/raising-livestock-zmaz79jazraw.

19.   Ibid.

20.   Ibid.

21.   Ibid.

CHAPTER 15—RAISING NATURAL, WHOLESOME, HOPE-FILLED CHILDREN

1.   Juliet Spurrier, "What Is Inside Those Disposable Diapers?," Baby Gear Lab, August 30, 2014, accessed May 15, 2017, https://www.babygearlab.com/expert-advice/what-is-inside-those-disposable-diapers.

2.   Ibid.

3.   Ibid.

4.   Julie Revelant, "Are Infant Cereals Really the Best First Food for Babies?," Fox News Health, September 11, 2016, accessed May 15, 2017, http://www.foxnews.com/health/2016/09/11/are-infant-cereals-really-best-first-food-for-babies.html.

5.   "Feeding Baby: How to Avoid Food Allergies," WebMD, accessed May 15, 2017, http://www.webmd.com/parenting/baby/baby-food-nutrition-9/introducing-new-foods.

6.   Sally Fallon, *Nourishing Traditions: The Cookbook That Challenges Politically Correct Nutrition and Diet Dictocrats* (Washington, DC: New Trends Publishing, 2001).

7.   Christine Carter, "Five Ways to Motivate Kids to Do Chores," *Parents*, accessed May 15, 2017, http://www.parents.com/kids/development/social/motivate-kids-to-do-chores/?.

8.   Joy Rynda, "How to Assign Age-Appropriate Chores to Children," *Children's Hospital of Wisconsin Blog*, May 4, 2017, accessed May 15, 2017, http://blog.chw.org/2017/05/how-to-assign-age-appropriate-chores-to-children/.

9.   Annie Stuart, "Divide and Conquer Household Chores," WebMD LLC, 2008, accessed June 6, 2017, http://www.webmd.com/parenting/features/chores-for-children#1; see also Kimberley Hibbert, "When to Start Your Kids on Chores," *Jamaica Observer*, November 17, 2014, accessed May 15, 2017, http://www.jamaicaobserver.com/magazines/allwoman/WHEN-TO-START-your-KIDS-on-chores_17916737?.

10.   Ibid.

11.   Ibid.

CHAPTER 16—NATURAL SOLUTIONS FOR CREATING ABUNDANCE

1.   "Free Download: EveryDollar Guide to Budgeting," *Dave Ramsey* (blog), accessed May 15, 2017, https://www.daveramsey.com/blog/free-download-budgeting-guide/.

2.   For more information, visit http://thepaleomama.com/paleo-meal-planning/.

3.   "Financial Peace: Your Money Made Simple," Dave Ramsey, accessed May 15, 2017, http://www.daveramsey.com/fpu/online.

4.   Jackie Ritz, "So You Wanna Start a Money Making Blog?," *The Paleo Mama* (blog), February 4, 2014, accessed May 15, 2017, http://thepaleomama.com/2014/02/wanna-start-money-making-blog/.

5.   Jackie Ritz, "How to Order dōTERRA Essential Oils," *The Paleo Mama* (blog), accessed May 15, 2017, http://thepaleomama.com/essential-oils/.

6.   "Are Credit Cards a Way of Life?," *Dave Ramsey* (blog), accessed May 15, 2017, http://www.daveramsey.com/blog/are-credit-cards-a-way-of-life/.

7.   "Seven Characteristics of Debt-Free People," *Dave Ramsey* (blog), accessed May 15, 2017, http://www.daveramsey.com/blog/7-characteristics-of-debt-free-people.

CONCLUSION—YOU CAN DO IT!

1.   "Helen Keller Quotes," BrainyQuote, accessed May 15, 2017, https://www.brainyquote.com/quotes/quotes/h/helenkelle114884.html.

INDEX

R

Ramsey, Dave 163–167, 169–170, 177
real food 19–25, 27–28, 31, 33–35, 38, 41, 47–49, 52, 56, 158
root cellar 125–127

S

shea butter 76, 95–97, 176
sheep 13, 29, 56, 143, 146, 159
silage 137
silicone-derived emollients 60
slow food 24
Smart Pots 12, 175
sodium lauryl (ether) sulfate (SLS, SLES) 60
spinosad 121
spirulina 70–71
stevia 23, 33–34, 64, 71, 75, 85
sulfate(s) 75

T

talc 60, 99,
toluene 61
triclosan 61, 104
turkey. *See* poultry
turmeric 81, 84–86

U

US Department of Agriculture's Hardiness Zone Map 12

W

weaning 156–158. See also *Nourishing Traditions*; Fallon, Sally

ABOUT THE AUTHOR

*J*ACKIE RITZ IS the founder and creator of the website *The Paleo Mama* (www.thepaleomama.com), where she has educated others on health and wellness for more than five years. Jackie and her husband have a ten-acre farm in western North Carolina, where they raise their two children and their many farm animals. Her love for growing things, raising things, and using natural ingredients from God's creation is what inspires her writing.

CONNECT WITH US!

CHARISMA HOUSE

(Spiritual Growth)

 Facebook.com/CharismaHouse

 @CharismaHouse

 Instagram.com/CharismaHouse

SILOAM

(Health)

 Pinterest.com/CharismaHouse

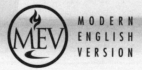

MODERN ENGLISH VERSION

(Bible)

www.mevbible.com